The Children's Hospital of Philadelphia
Guide to Asthma

The Children's
Hospital of
Philadelphia
Guide to Asthma

How to Help Your Child
Live a Healthier Life

Edited by
Julian Lewis Allen, M.D.
Tyra Bryant-Stephens, M.D.
Nicholas A. Pawlowski, M.D.
with
Sheila Buff and Martha M. Jablow

WILEY
John Wiley & Sons, Inc.

Published by John Wiley & Sons, Inc., Hoboken, New Jersey
Published simultaneously in Canada

Design and production by Navta Associates, Inc.

The information contained in this book is not intended to serve as a replacement for professional medical advice. Any use of the information in this book is at the reader's discretion. The author and the publisher specifically disclaim any and all liability arising directly or indirectly from the use or application of any information contained in this book. A health care professional should be consulted regarding your specific situation.

For general information about our other products and services, please contact our Customer Care Department within the United States at (800) 762-2974, outside the United States at (317) 572-3993 or fax (317) 572-4002.

Wiley also publishes its books in a variety of electronic formats. Some content that appears in print may not be available in electronic books. For more information about Wiley products, visit our web site at www.wiley.com.

Library of Congress Cataloging-in-Publication Data:
The Children's Hospital of Philadelphia guide to asthma : how to help your child live a healthier life / edited by Julian Lewis Allen . . . [et al].
    p.   cm.
Includes index.
    ISBN 0-471-44116-3 (paper)
1. Asthma in children. 2. Asthma in children—Treatment. I. Allen, Julian Lewis.
RJ436.A68 C48 2004
618.92'238—dc22
                                                                        2003025750

Printed in the United States of America

10 9 8 7 6 5 4 3 2 1

Contents

Preface

This book was conceived by physicians and nurse practitioners who care for infants, children, and adolescents with asthma at The Children's Hospital of Philadelphia. Our objective was to produce a practical book for parents and caregivers that clearly explains asthma and its management. We also wished to emphasize our philosophy that, with proper education and treatment, nearly all children with asthma should be able to participate in all the same activities as other children. Asthma is an illness that is not to be feared, but respected, understood, and acted upon.

Your child's pediatrician, family doctor, or asthma specialist may not strictly adhere to all the specific recommendations in this book, but that does not mean they are treating your child incorrectly. No two practitioners approach things in exactly the same way. This book should, however, be a useful starting point for discussion with your child's asthma care provider about why he or she is prescribing the treatment and the reasoning behind the management plan.

In this book, you will find a series of vignettes about children with asthma. You may even recognize descriptions of symptoms similar to those of your child. You will also find at the end of this book a Resources section with "tools" that can be copied and used in the day-to-day management of your child's asthma. We hope you find these vignettes and tools useful in increasing your understanding of asthma and the role that its management can play in helping your child achieve a happy, fulfilling childhood that is as free from asthma symptoms as possible.

—J. L. A

—T. B.-S.

—N. A. P.

Authorship and Acknowledgments

The creation of this book has been a team effort by health care professionals who treat children with asthma at The Children's Hospital of Philadelphia. They include:

Senior Editors and Authors
Julian Lewis Allen, M.D.
Chief, Division of Pulmonary Medicine and Cystic Fibrosis Center
Robert Girard Morse Endowed Chair in Pulmonary Medicine
The Children's Hospital of Philadelphia
Professor of Pediatrics, University of Pennsylvania School of Medicine

Tyra Bryant Stephens, M.D., F.A.A.P.
Medical Director, Community Asthma Prevention Program
The Children's Hospital of Philadelphia
Clinical Assistant Professor of Pediatrics, University of Pennsylvania
    School of Medicine

Nicholas A. Pawlowski, M.D.
Allergy Section Chief, Division of Allergy and Immunology,
The Children's Hospital of Philadelphia
Associate Professor of Pediatrics, University of Pennsylvania School of
    Medicine

Contributing Authors

Janet L. Beausoleil, M.D.
Attending Physician, Allergy Section
Division of Allergy and Immunology
The Children's Hospital of Philadelphia
Clinical Assistant Professor of Pediatrics, University of Pennsylvania
School of Medicine

Robin C. Capecci, M.S.W., L.S.W
Medical Social Worker
The Children's Hospital of Philadelphia

Russell G. Clayton, Sr., D.O.
Director, Asthma Program
Division of Pulmonary Medicine
Medical Director, Pulmonary Function Laboratory
The Children's Hospital of Philadelphia
Assistant Professor of Pediatrics, University of Pennsylvania School of
Medicine

Joel Fiedler, M.D.
Attending Physician, Division of Allergy and Immunology
The Children's Hospital of Philadelphia
Clinical Assistant Professor of Pediatrics, University of Pennsylvania
School of Medicine

Jonathan M. Spergel, M.D., Ph.D.
Attending Physician, Division of Allergy and Immunology
The Children's Hospital of Philadelphia
Assistant Professor of Pediatrics, University of Pennsylvania School of
Medicine

Marcia Winston, M.S.N., R.N., C.P.N.P., AE-C
Certified Pediatric Nurse Practitioner
Certified Asthma Educator
Coordinator, Asthma Program

Division of Pulmonary Medicine
The Children's Hospital of Philadelphia

Joseph J. Zorc, M.D.
Attending Physician, Division of Emergency Medicine
The Children's Hospital of Philadelphia
Assistant Professor of Pediatrics and Emergency Medicine
University of Pennsylvania School of Medicine

Their efforts were assisted by freelance writers Sheila Buff and Martha M. Jablow. Illustrations by Marie Garafano were made possible through a grant from The Pew Charitable Trusts. The initial idea to publish this book originated with now-retired Children's Hospital Vice President Shirley Bonnem, who has guided from preparation to publication this and nine other books for parents and caregivers.

Introduction

It is more than a decade since The Children's Hospital of Philadelphia was invited to publish a book for parents entitled *The Children's Hospital of Philadelphia: A Parent's Guide to Allergies and Asthma*. Much has happened since that book came out. The incidence of asthma continues to rise dramatically not only in the United States but also around the world. Ten years ago, the Centers for Disease Control and Prevention (CDC) estimated that approximately 3 million children under the age of 18 suffered from asthma. Today, the number has risen by almost two-thirds to 4.8 million children with asthma. The mortality rate of the pediatric population with asthma increased 55.6 percent between 1979 and 1998.

Asthma is not to be taken lightly. When untreated, it not only causes children difficulty breathing, but it also lands many in emergency rooms and hospitals and costs parents countless lost time from work because they must take their children to medical appointments or keep them home from school.

This pattern can be reversed. With better understanding of symptoms, their causes, and correct medications that prevent and treat symptoms, parents can help their children enjoy a healthier, more active life. That is the point of this book. It is intended to enable parents, caregivers, and young patients to improve the management of asthma.

This book contains not only the most up-to-date information relating to the illness but also techniques that enable families to manage asthma by understanding conditions that trigger the problem and infections that may compound it. The goal is to learn how to cope with this chronic

1

condition in a way that permits children with asthma to lead lives that are as normal as possible. The book's sixteen chapters discuss what asthma is, getting it under control, managing an episode of the disease, asthma emergencies, toddlers and teenagers with asthma, sports and exercise, asthma when the child is away from home, and asthma and the health care system. A list of community and national resources and an index are included, as well.

The book was in part conceived as a result of a grant from The Pew Charitable Trusts to The Children's Hospital of Philadelphia. One purpose of this grant was to help integrate the care of children with asthma across the large tri-state Children's Hospital pediatric network, and to foster communication among the many sites where children with asthma receive care. These include the offices of primary care physicians or pediatricians, pulmonology and allergy specialists, and emergency departments within hospitals. In addition, the grant enabled the authors of this book, who are Children's Hospital doctors and nurse practitioners who care for children with asthma, to formulate many of the suggestions you will read on these pages. They are applicable to patients everywhere.

I cannot help but compare the technological advances of today with the limited ones available during my early years at The Children's Hospital of Philadelphia when the late Harold I. Lecks, M.D., developed a program for children with allergies and asthma. Both conditions had become ordinary enough at that time to mandate a special service for children. Among his many achievements in that particular field, Dr. Lecks led a vigorous collaborative effort that included anesthesiology, pharmacology, psychiatry, and rehabilitative medicine. One of the results was the creation by allergists and anesthesiologists of a clinical asthma scoring system that has been used extensively in pediatrics. Contributions like these by dedicated health professionals continue to improve the lives of children with asthma and allergies today.

—C. Everett Koop, M.D., Sc. D.
Surgeon-in-Chief Emeritus, The Children's Hospital of Philadelphia
Former Surgeon General, United States Public Health Service

1

When Your Child Has Asthma

As a mother holds her seven-month-old baby, she notices that he's breathing faster and harder than normal. With each breath, his belly is moving in and out more than usual. She hears a faint "whistling" sound with each breath as well. She never saw this in her older child. "What's wrong?" she worries.

The father of an eight-year-old observes that his daughter often gets winded when she plays outside. She slows down and sits on a bench while her friends race around the playground.

A twelve-year-old has trouble inhaling enough air. He describes the sensation as "trying to suck in air through a soda straw."

These children have asthma, the most common chronic health problem among children today. *Chronic* means that the condition is ongoing—it comes and goes but never disappears entirely. Does asthma mean that your child will have a lifetime of serious, continual health problems? *Absolutely not.*

Asthma cannot be cured, but it can be treated and controlled. Your child can lead a normal, active life. Bringing asthma under control may not happen overnight. It will take some effort by you, your child, and the people around you, but there is no question that children with asthma can be helped. The purpose of this book is to help parents and children limit the frequency and severity of asthma symptoms by controlling environmental factors that trigger symptoms and by managing medicines that prevent and treat asthma episodes.

If your child has been diagnosed with asthma—or if you suspect it— you want to understand as much as possible about its causes, treatments, and prognosis so you can help your child manage this disease without compromising all the joys and adventures of childhood. The more you learn about asthma, the more confident you will be about helping your child avoid serious consequences and medical emergencies. Children have a great talent for picking up parents' vibes, so the more knowledgeable and assured you are about controlling your child's asthma, the more at ease your child will be.

This chapter will give you a general overview of asthma. Let's begin with some basic facts:

- Nearly 5 million American children have asthma, and the numbers are growing nationally and worldwide.

- Over 7 percent (about one in fifteen) of children between ages five and fourteen have asthma. That's up from only 3 percent in the 1980s.

- Asthma is the leading reason why children miss school, visit emergency rooms, and are hospitalized, as well as a major reason why parents miss work because they must care for children with asthma.

JUST WHAT IS ASTHMA?

Asthma is a chronic disorder that swells the walls of the lungs' airways. As the airways swell, the muscles around them tighten, squeezing the airways. At the same time, the airways clog with mucus. These combined factors—swelling, tightening, squeezing, and mucus—keep air from moving in and out of the lungs as easily as it should. That's why your child coughs, wheezes, or has trouble breathing.

This doesn't mean that all children with asthma have the same symptoms or have them all the time. Some never cough. Others rarely wheeze. Some show symptoms only when they are physically active, or have colds, or during seasons when allergies trigger wheezing, coughing, or difficulty breathing.

Asthma is always present but not always observable. When symptoms kick up, we call it an asthma *flare*. Some medical professionals also call it an asthma episode, attack, or exacerbation. If you want to know what a flare feels like, take a breath and hold it for a few seconds. Without breathing out, take another breath, and then another and another. You'll soon be able to take only very shallow breaths. Your chest will feel quite full and even painful. You may feel like you're choking. You may also start to feel a little panicky. Imagine feeling that way and also having to cough uncontrollably. Now you have a better understanding of how unpleasant and frightening a severe asthma attack can be for your child.

ASTHMA AND THE LUNGS

Doctors and nurses refer to the swelling of the airways as *inflammation* and the squeezing of the airways as *bronchospasm* or *bronchoconstriction* of the muscles that encircle the airways. What is the cause? To answer that, here is a quick lesson in how the lungs work:

The lungs' major job is to bring oxygen into the bloodstream and remove carbon dioxide from it. As you inhale through your nose and mouth, air enters your windpipe, or *trachea*. Picture your airways as an upside-down tree with the windpipe as the trunk. The windpipe goes down your throat and branches out at the top of your chest into two large tubes or *bronchi,* with one *bronchus* for each lung.

Within each lung, the main bronchus divides to form several smaller tubes that branch again and again to form hundreds of thousands of even smaller tubes called *bronchioles*. The bronchioles split off into millions of pockets of tiny air sacs called *alveoli*. Your lungs have over 300 million alveoli. These air sacs resemble tiny clusters of grapes at the end of each bronchiole branch. Within the air sacs, life-giving oxygen from the air you inhale is exchanged for carbon dioxide, the waste product that leaves your body when you breathe out.

Inhaled air often contains harmful things like dust and bacteria. Your nose, windpipe, and bronchial tubes have several defenses to keep these nasty irritants from reaching your lungs. Airways are lined with membranes that produce mucus, the slippery, sticky substance that traps tiny particles and keeps them from getting inhaled any deeper into the lungs. Airways are also lined with tiny hairs that gently sweep the mucus-trapped particles up and out. Coughing is another defense. When you cough, you force air and mucus out of your lungs along with any trapped particles.

Sometimes particles can sneak past the first line of defense and go deeper into the bronchial tubes. In an effort to get rid of them, the body

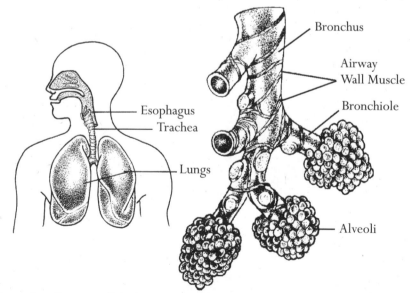

Figure 1.   Structure of the lung.

reacts with inflammation. Cells in the airways' lining release substances that make the lining swell, produce more mucus, and make the muscles around the bronchial tubes tighten and squeeze the tubes. Airway swelling and tightening happen to just about everybody at times. That's what makes you cough when you have a bad cold or flu or when you breathe in smoke or other irritants.

Children with asthma have highly sensitive airways. They usually have a little swelling in their airways all the time. Your child can't feel it, and you can't see it happening in your child. This is sometimes called "silent asthma." When a youngster with asthma inhales something that affects her breathing tubes, like pollen or cigarette smoke, her sensitive airways overreact. The tubes swell more and fill with mucus, the muscles tighten, and the child coughs and wheezes as she struggles to breathe. Doctors and nurses sometimes say that children with asthma

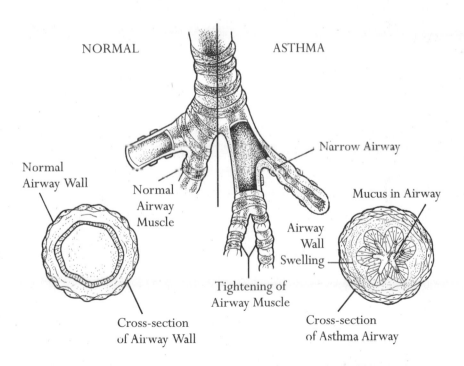

Figure 2.   A normal airway (left) and an airway showing signs of asthma (right).

have "twitchy," "hyperreactive," or "hyperresponsive" airways, because they react severely and for a long time to substances in the air that usually don't bother other people.

Why does the asthmatic lung respond this way? To the best of our current knowledge, the immune system is the cause. When an irritant like pollen is inhaled, for example, chemicals in the pollen are released into the lung and cause swelling, muscle tightening, and overproduction of mucus. But this rarely occurs just once. With each new exposure to an infection or an irritant (or "trigger") that causes even the mildest allergy flare, inflammatory cells increase the reaction, making it stronger and last longer.

When scientists look under the microscope, they see that the invading cells of inflammation are scattered throughout the airways. Imagine the lungs of a child who either keeps getting respiratory infections or breathes in allergy triggers over and over again. The airway inflammation builds up to higher and higher levels, and asthma flares become more difficult to control. Symptoms are more intense. They last longer and are harder to control with medicines.

ASTHMA TRIGGERS

Anything that affects the airways of a child with asthma is called a trigger. It is often something your child is allergic to, such as pollen or dust mites (tiny "bugs" that live in carpet or fabrics), as well as irritants like cigarette smoke. Exposure to a trigger—even in very small amounts—can set off a flare or sudden worsening of asthma symptoms. (The connection between allergies and asthma will be discussed in chapter 3.)

Asthma flares are also commonly triggered by colds, exercise, or exposure to cold, dry air, as on a winter day. Respiratory infections are the most common triggers for flares in children. Usually these are common viruses that are "only a cold" in other children who don't have asthma. For them, the cough is not the same, and they don't develop the other features of asthma described previously.

Upper respiratory tract infections (common colds) caused by viruses usually produce a runny nose before coughing or other symptoms begin. But not all of the time. If you watch carefully, you will find that not every runny nose and respiratory infection will cause an asthma flare. Thank goodness! A child who is only triggered by viral infections will recover completely between asthma flares.

Unfortunately, viral infections can occur frequently. A child might get a new one even before completely recovering from an asthma flare. When this happens, it seems as if the child continues being sick for an unusually long time. A cold usually should last a week or less, but if the cold triggers an asthma flare, the cough may hang on longer. Before you know it, the child catches another cold. Tracking nighttime cough or other symptoms will help you sort out what is really happening. When night symptoms appear, disappear, and then return again, a second flare is quite likely.

When a child's asthma is triggered only by respiratory infections, a typical pattern of symptoms appears over the course of a year. First there is a flare, then complete recovery, and later additional flares at random intervals. During the winter months, a child may have many flares, but if there is time to recover, all asthma symptoms will disappear between the attacks.

This has important implications for treatment. If your child has no symptoms for a long time and no flares, it might seem correct *not* to give medicines every day. You are right! But if the flares come often, perhaps every week or two, your child may need daily medicine to help prevent frequent flares. (More about this will be given in chapter 5.)

Allergy triggers can be found indoors and out. A child may be continually exposed to allergy triggers, including dust mites or animal dander from pets in your home. (*Dander* refers to flakes of skin or dried saliva from animals with fur or feathers.) If a child is sensitive to pollens, she may be exposed to them not only when she's outdoors but also indoors if the windows are kept open—and especially if window fans are used.

Children may have intermittent exposure to allergy triggers too. A child who is allergic or "sensitized" to animal dander, for example, may be exposed only while visiting a friend's home where a furry pet lives.

Brief exposure—just a few hours—to a trigger can cause symptoms and even a flare if a child is very sensitive. But allergy-triggered flares will be shorter than an attack brought on by a virus, which typically lasts about a week or longer.

Important fact: Daily exposure to allergy triggers inside a home will cause increased airway inflammation. If the exposure continues for months, the inflammation builds, and so do the symptoms. Problems like seasonal pollen exposure can also create prolonged symptoms. These seasonal patterns last only as long as the pollen season lasts, of course.

When a child is exposed to allergy triggers daily throughout the year, it is called a perennial problem. The greater the number of significant triggers, the more likely there will be constant or repeated exposure. And increased exposures mean increased risk for chronic inflammation in the lungs. As exposures increase, so does airway inflammation. And daily symptoms follow close behind.

It's important to understand that all exposures—both allergy triggers and infections—pile up on one another. While the presence of one trigger alone may not produce obvious symptoms, several combined triggers may do so. A child who has lots of triggers and persistent symptoms will have a more difficult time when a viral infection sparks a new flare that may be more severe and take longer to abate.

Constant inflammation in the lungs caused by allergy exposures makes it easier for viral infections to bring on flares. For example:

> Katie is allergic to cats, but her family doesn't want to give away
> their cat. They try to keep it away from Katie, and it sleeps in her
> brother's room. But Katie has more virus-triggered asthma attacks
> than her friend Sandy, another cat-allergic child, who isn't fre-
> quently inhaling cat dander.

Irritants are a common problem. Exposures may be intermittent or ongoing, almost every day. Tobacco smoke is the classic culprit in this category. Even if parents step outdoors to smoke, they bring tobacco fumes into the home on their clothing. This passive or indirect exposure can cause problems for infants and children of all ages. You may think that's unlikely or far-fetched, but the by-products of tobacco smoke can be detected in a child's bloodstream, which proves that the transfer occurs even when tobacco is smoked out-of-doors. Children with high levels of tobacco chemicals in their blood have been proven to have much greater problems with asthma.

Other types of smoke—from fireplaces, wood-burning stoves, candles, or incense—and fumes from cleaning products or perfumes are also irritants. They're worse during the winter. When doors and windows are closed, it's difficult for a child to escape these irritants. Long-term exposure to large amounts of irritants and can create more inflammation in a child's lungs. As the number of irritants increases, the inflammation and symptoms build. And flares occur more often.

Certain medicines may also trigger asthma symptoms in a susceptible patient, but this does not happen often. Examples are drugs used to treat high blood pressure (angiotensin converting enzyme inhibitors) or migraine (beta-blockers), aspirin, and nonsteroidal anti-inflammatory drugs (NSAIDs, like ibuprofen).

When a child is evaluated for asthma, physicians and nurse practitioners will carefully consider all the triggers that increase the inflammation level in the lungs as well as other conditions that can complicate asthma.

By decreasing your child's exposure to triggers, you can do a great deal to reduce the number and severity of flares. This isn't always easy, but as you'll learn in later chapters, some triggers can be eliminated or reduced very simply. Others may take more effort. But with each step you take to remove or reduce triggers, you'll see benefits—an improvement in your child's symptoms, and fewer medicines will be needed to control them.

RECOGNIZING ASTHMA SYMPTOMS

Asthma is a highly individual condition. Symptoms can range from very mild to severe and even life threatening. Symptoms may appear only occasionally and last for just a little while. Or they may occur daily to several times a week and become more severe. They may even go from mild to severe in a short time. No two children with asthma are alike, but the main symptoms of asthma include:

Coughing. One of the main symptoms of asthma is typically a dry cough that becomes worse at night, often to the point of waking a child. Parents have also described the cough as deep, wet, junky, barky, croupy, and seal-like.

Wheezing. The classic asthma symptom is wheezing—a hoarse, high-pitched whistling or squeaky noise as a child breathes in and out. Wheezing tends to get worse at night.

Shortness of breath or rapid breathing. Sometimes parents of children with asthma describe this as heavy breathing. Because he is short of breath, your child may slow down and stop playing. He might also get tired, irritable, or become uninterested in things around him.

Chest tightness. Young children may say their chests hurt or "feel funny." Older children may describe the sensation as tight or achy, or they may say they have chest pain and feel like a weight is sitting on their chest.

Most children with asthma start showing symptoms before they are five years old. At one time, doctors thought that children under age three didn't get asthma, but today we know that children as young as six months can have asthma. Symptoms in very young children are similar to those in older ones—coughing, wheezing, rapid breathing, and fatigue. A baby can't tell you her chest feels tight, of course, but you might notice that she has problems feeding or makes grunting noises when sucking or breathing. Her nostrils may also flare as she works harder to breathe.

As you'll learn in chapter 2, children with asthma should be diagnosed as early as possible. Early diagnosis means they will start receiving the treatment needed to keep them thriving and active and to prevent colds from turning into asthma flares. Early diagnosis and treatment can also help their lungs develop normally and reach full capacity, which may help them avoid developing breathing problems when they are adults.

Asthma Flares— Mild, Moderate, Severe

Asthma symptoms can be so mild that you might not even realize your child has them—until the symptoms suddenly become worse. Then you'll realize in a hurry that your child is having an asthma flare.

During a mild flare, a child has a little trouble breathing. She breathes a bit faster than usual. She may be a little short of breath and wheezy, especially when she exhales. She may also have some coughing, but she's alert and able to talk easily. If she has a cold with a cough, you might not even notice that she's having an asthma flare.

If the flare is moderate, all the breathing symptoms will be worse. The wheezing will be much more noticeable. It will be louder as she breathes out. She won't be able to get enough breath to talk easily. You'll probably notice that the muscles between her ribs move in and out as she struggles to breathe. You may also notice that it takes her much longer to breathe out than to breathe in.

If the asthma attack is severe, breathing will be very difficult. She'll wheeze and cough severely, won't be able to talk, and will be so short of breath that she uses the muscles of her neck, chest, and abdomen to breathe. Her skin color, lips, or nail beds may look quite pale or even bluish. If the attack is very severe, so little air will be moving in and out of her lungs that she won't even wheeze.

A severe asthma attack is a medical emergency. Call for an ambulance or take your child to an emergency room at once.

Even a moderate flare is a highly upsetting experience for a child—and for you—and may mean a trip to the emergency room or a hospitalization. Fortunately for you and your child, asthma flares don't have to be this bad.

The Key to Treatment

Control of airway inflammation is the key to successful asthma treatment. To control inflammation in the lungs, there are two main things to do:

First, control your child's environment the best you can. Exposure to viral infections or colds is inevitable among children (although good frequent hand washing can help prevent the spread of colds). But many allergy and irritant triggers can be controlled effectively. Please remember: controlling these triggers may help reduce the need for medicine.

Second, use controller or anti-inflammatory medicines. Based on the pattern of your child's asthma symptoms, your physician or nurse practitioner may prescribe daily medicine to keep the asthma under control. The minimum effective doses and the safest medicines will be tailored specifically for your child. (More about medicines will be given in chapter 5.)

TREATMENT GOALS

If you work toward these two goals, you can learn and achieve the important tasks for successful asthma care:

1. Your child should reach a "baseline," a period of time in which no symptoms appear. Between flares, your child should have normal lung function (determined by a special breathing test called spirometry, described on pages 26–27) and no symptoms.
2. You and your child can effectively control flares by learning when and how to treat symptoms as soon as they appear. The goal is to decrease three things: the number of flares, the severity of symptoms during the flares, and the length of time your child is sick. This will mean less lost sleep for child and parent and less downtime from school and work.

In chapter 7 we will discuss a written "asthma management plan" for increasing medicines to relieve your child's symptoms when they arise. For the moment, just keep in mind that the keys to controlling asthma are sticking with such plans and recognizing new flares at their very beginning. If you do so, the number of flares will decrease, and they will be easier to get through.

ASTHMA MEDICINES

Today a large array of safe, effective medicines are available to control asthma and treat flares. Two basic types of medicines are used to control asthma:

Controller medicines provide long-term control of asthma by decreasing lung inflammation and its symptoms. The classic example is a steroid inhaler. Controller medicines are given regularly, usually on a daily basis, to prevent symptoms and flares. They do *not* bring immediate relief from symptoms and are not intended to do so.

Quick-relief medicines are taken when symptoms like cough and shortness of breath first appear. The classic example of this type is albuterol or related medicines (Maxair or Xopenex). These medicines treat asthma symptoms but do not decrease airway inflammation. In other words, they only treat the symptoms but not the cause of asthma. However, they are very effective when asthma symptoms get worse.

If a child needs quick-relief medicine on a regular basis, you can conclude that airway inflammation is out of control. Asthma specialists today believe that if a child needs albuterol more than once a week or uses more than two canisters a year, his asthma is not under good control. Instead, daily anti-inflammatory medicines are needed to control the airway inflammation.

Once a child's asthma is under good control with the right medicines, flares don't have to occur at all. You'll learn a lot more in chapters 4, 5, and 6 about how an individual treatment plan and the right medicines can bring your child's asthma under control. Other chapters of this book will help you learn ways to manage asthma flares and help avoid them.

THE ROOTS OF ASTHMA

Triggers set off asthma flares, but they are not the reason your child has asthma in the first place. What is the cause? There's no single answer to that question at this time, but asthma has several suspected sources.

Family history is probably one major reason for asthma. If relatives have asthma or allergies, a child has a good chance of having them as well. The chances of this are even greater when a child inherits the tendency toward asthma and allergies from both sides of the family. A family history of asthma doesn't guarantee that a child will have it, though. Many children with asthma have no known family history.

Low-birth-weight children are more likely to have asthma than heavier newborns. In younger children, asthma is more common in boys than girls. Girls are more likely to get it when they reach puberty. By adolescence, the number of boys and girls with asthma equals out.

Allergies, which are immune system reactions to substances such as pollen or dust mites, play a central role in asthma. In fact, the majority of children with asthma have allergies. But not all children with allergies have asthma. If you can identify your child's allergies and get them under control, you'll be able to help bring her asthma under control (see chapter 3).

Your child's environment may be part of why he has asthma. Cigarette smoke, as mentioned earlier, is a major preventable asthma trigger. In some cases, it not only triggers asthma but also causes it. Children who live with a smoker are about 25 percent more likely to have asthma than youngsters who live in nonsmoking homes. A woman's smoking during pregnancy makes it about twice as likely that her baby will later develop asthma.

Today's children spend most of their time indoors—in well-insulated houses and schools with carpets, upholstered furniture, drapes, other dust collectors, and dust mites. In urban neighborhoods with substandard housing, children are exposed to additional triggers, such as air pollution and cockroaches. This could be one reason why asthma rates are higher in city neighborhoods than in suburban areas. When a child's inherited tendency toward asthma is combined with other environmental risks, the chances of having asthma increase.

Some interesting theories exist about why people get asthma. Worldwide, the number of people with asthma has been climbing rapidly, especially in industrialized nations. Some researchers think that the jump in asthma cases in these countries could have something to do with the decrease in childhood illnesses, such as measles, and the over-all increase in cleanliness (from using antibacterial soaps, lotions, and cleaning products, for example). According to this thinking, the body uses two types of immunity. One fights bacteria and viruses, while the other helps fight off parasites, such as intestinal worms. This parasite-fighting part of the immune system is also responsible for causing allergies. Exposure to bacteria and viruses actually *helps* a child's immune system develop properly by "training" it to recognize and attack those harmful germs. When children live in a cleaner environment and don't get sick as often, the part of their immune system that fights germs doesn't have much to do. With no bacteria or viruses to battle, the immune system becomes more active on the parasite-fighting/allergy side. Certain genes have been linked to asthma, and some of them are more common in countries with high rates of parasitic infections.

WHAT *DOESN'T* CAUSE ASTHMA?

Researchers cannot say for certain exactly what causes asthma, but they can rule out some old suspects. Not too long ago, asthma was thought to have a psychological cause. Today we know that asthma is definitely not psychosomatic, or "all in the child's head." Children with asthma have a real medical problem. It isn't something they dream up or bring on just to get attention or to avoid going to school. A child with untreated asthma may not feel well much of the time and may need considerable parental attention, but the attention he seeks isn't the cause of asthma. Likewise, asthma isn't caused by a parent's overprotectiveness or over-involvement with a child.

Children today receive many shots to protect them against serious childhood illnesses such as measles, whooping cough, and polio. Vaccination shots do not cause asthma or make it worse. If your child has asthma, discuss her immunization or vaccination schedule with your doctor. Some shots shouldn't be given while a child is taking certain medicines or if she has egg allergies.

Outgrowing Asthma

One of the biggest myths about asthma is that most children "just grow out of it." This isn't actually the case. A minority of children with asthma will leave asthma behind as they grow older. They generally had only mild asthma in early childhood and usually don't have allergies. As they grow, their airways become larger, and they stop wheezing and having other asthma symptoms.

An important research study followed a group of children from birth to age six. They were monitored carefully for all respiratory symptoms. They also had careful allergy evaluations and specialized lung function testing, beginning at birth. The study found that approximately 40 percent of these children coughed and/or wheezed at least a couple times during their first six years of life. Pretty common problems!

Among the group of children who had respiratory symptoms, one-third had trouble beginning within their first year of life, but those problems disappeared by age three. These were children with "smaller lungs," and their symptoms were due to viral infections. They didn't have asthma and had no long-term problems. This is why many health professionals will not attach a label of asthma to a child (especially a baby or a toddler) unless he or she has repeated episodes for a year or more. This is a wise decision, but asthma medicines should not be withheld if they have been found to help the child, even if it is not yet certain that the child will develop asthma.

Another third of these children will start to show asthma symptoms early, in their first three years, and continue to have repeated episodes of wheezing and coughing as they get older. These children have asthma. The remaining group of children who had no trouble during their first two or three years of life, but began symptoms later, also have asthma. This group is especially prone to allergy and environmental triggers that create airway inflammation.

Over time, some children can be expected to see their asthma improve.

Those who have repeated viral infections during their first ten years of life will slowly begin to have fewer problems with flares created by viral infections. Those with persistent symptoms—signs of airway inflammation ongoing every day—will continue to have increasing amounts of airway inflammation or problems if their environmental exposures are not eliminated. They may need medicines every day as well.

As children get older, they may go through long periods when asthma seems to get better on its own. A child who had asthma problems in his early years, but then improved, is still at risk for some difficulties in adult life. A classic example is the adult who begins to have difficulties in his thirties and forties after a long stretch without any asthma symptoms. He may have even forgotten his childhood asthma problems. That's another important reason for careful, accurate diagnosis early in life followed by a thorough treatment plan that includes regular checkups and lung function testing. Once they're old enough, all children with asthma should learn to recognize symptoms whenever they occur and know how to treat them or seek help.

Doctors cannot predict exactly which children will grow out of asthma and which won't. In general, the milder and less frequent the symptoms, the more likely a child will outgrow it. If your child has more severe asthma along with allergies and a family history of asthma, the chances of outgrowing it aren't as good.

PARTNERING WITH YOUR CHILD'S HEALTH PROFESSIONAL

The best advice is simple and straightforward: work with your child's physician or nurse practitioner to review the pattern of illness that you have observed over the last six months. Ask yourself questions like these: How often do symptoms occur? What triggers the symptoms? How often do flares occur? It's also helpful to keep a diary of symptoms, how long they last, what season or time of day they occur, how they were treated, how long it took to end the flare, etc.

From your observations, and in consultation with your child's doctor or nurse practitioner, make a plan for controlling the environment and for adjusting asthma medicines for the next six months. Update and adjust the plan regularly. There is no one-size-fits-all answer here. Some children may need to see a doctor more frequently than every six months, while others may need to be seen less often. Only over time will you gain a clear idea of your individual child's pattern of illness. It may improve with time or even seem to disappear. As we'll discuss in chapter 5, long-term controller medicines are offered based on the pattern of illness, not on single episodes, so it's important that you have a clear understanding of your child's pattern.

Too many children see a medical professional only when they're ill. But it's important to make follow-up visits when your child is well. When you and your child go to a medical appointment, ask questions and expect information. This is especially important when a child is well because this is a good time to review how to recognize symptoms and gain assurance about how to treat them. Medicines can be decreased if your child is symptom-free and lung function is normal.

Lung-function testing during these healthy periods is important because it can confirm that a child is doing well, sometimes even after medicines are decreased or stopped. Silent problems may also be detected. Although a child seems symptom-free, there may be decreases in her lung function. Without this knowledge, appropriate medicines may not be given. Don't fall into the trap of stopping your child's asthma medicines because she "seems fine." The child may be well *because* of the asthma medicines. Discuss all medicine changes with your physician or nurse practitioner first.

In the end, you will learn that your child is improving thanks to all your hard work in controlling the environment, recognizing symptoms, and providing medicine every day and during flares. You will continue to learn more about asthma and feel more assured about medicines and the use of your child's asthma management plan.

All of us who treat children with asthma at The Children's Hospital of Philadelphia hope that this book will be an important step in your understanding of asthma and will provide useful tools to control it. It is important for parents and older children to become active partners with their medical professionals. Continue to learn about asthma!

2

Diagnosing Asthma

Finding out if your child has asthma isn't always easy. There's no one simple medical test for asthma, so the diagnosis depends on a child's overall *pattern* of symptoms. For that reason, it's important for parents to notice a variety of signs and symptoms that combine to form a pattern. If you suspect asthma, make an appointment with your child's doctor, take notes about the symptom patterns you've observed, and share them with the doctor.

IS IT REALLY ASTHMA?

Asthma is a common reason for wheezing and other breathing problems in children, but it's not the only one. Many common childhood illnesses can make a child cough, wheeze, and have trouble breathing. To complicate matters, colds and other upper respiratory illnesses are asthma triggers.

One or two episodes of wheezing in combination with a respiratory infection are common among young children, but this doesn't always mean asthma. With younger children especially, a doctor might decide that the wheezing and coughing are just from a bad cold or perhaps from a virus that causes bronchitis (inflammation of medium-size airways) or bronchiolitis (inflammation of the smaller airways). One such virus is called respiratory syncytial virus (RSV), but other viruses can cause wheezing as well. About half of all infants and toddlers who wheeze when they get colds will outgrow it.

Doctors tend to under-diagnose asthma in young children for two reasons: (1) many youngsters do outgrow wheezing from colds; and (2) some children have severe asthma symptoms while they have a cold but don't show any symptoms when they're well. Under-diagnosis is a problem because early detection of asthma is important. The sooner asthma is diagnosed, the sooner treatment can begin. Treatment not only makes a child feel better, but it may also help keep the asthma from becoming more severe or even causing permanent lung damage.

Wheezing with a cold is a sign that a child *might* have asthma. Don't ignore the warning. If your child has mild wheezing once or twice with a cold but recovers quickly and stops coughing and wheezing as soon as he starts to feel better, the symptoms probably were caused by the cold. It's not unusual for a child to have frequent colds—one a month or even more often is normal. A cold generally lasts for just a few days, and a child returns to normal quickly when it's over. Recurrent wheezing with colds, however, is not normal and may mean a child has asthma.

Consider these patterns:

- If your child has frequent colds that last for a week or longer each time,
- If your child wheezes with each cold, or
- If your child seems to have just one long cold with continuous coughing, then asthma could be the underlying problem.

Similarly, if your child is diagnosed with a respiratory infection, such as bronchitis or bronchiolitis, more than once or twice in a year, asthma could be the culprit. Repeated bouts of coughing and wheezing, with or without an upper respiratory infection, are almost always due to asthma.

There's a saying in medicine, however, that "all that wheezes is not asthma." Sometimes a child's health problem is diagnosed as asthma when it really isn't. A foreign object—a coin, a small piece of carrot or peanut—stuck in the child's lower airways can cause coughing or wheezing. A number of other diseases, such as cystic fibrosis, heart disease, and certain immune deficiencies can also seem like asthma. If that's the case, the symptoms won't get better when the child is treated for asthma, and it will soon be clear that asthma isn't the underlying problem.

Other medical conditions sometimes can make asthma worse. One example is gastroesophageal reflux disease (GERD), in which stomach acid regurgitates back up the esophagus (the tube between the mouth and stomach) and may spill over into the airways. That irritates the airways and causes inflammation and bronchospasm.

STEPS IN MAKING THE DIAGNOSIS

Medical history: The first and most important step in accurately diagnosing asthma is a careful, complete medical history. Your child's doctor will start by asking a lot of questions about your family history of allergy and asthma. The tendency to have allergies and asthma often runs in families. Among at least half of all children with asthma, one or both parents (more likely the mother) have allergies or asthma. Children who have already been diagnosed with allergy symptoms, such as eczema (skin rash) or rhinitis (runny nose), or with a food allergy, are more likely to have asthma as well. (You'll learn more about the asthma and allergy connection in the next chapter.)

Symptom patterns: The doctor or nurse practitioner will ask you and your child for a lot of details about the child's shortness of breath, coughing, wheezing, and chest tightness. These questions are an important first step in understanding the child's symptom pattern:

- Does your child cough and wheeze year-round or just during certain times of the year?
- Does she have at least some symptoms, such as slight wheezing, all the time? Do the symptoms go away and then flare up again?
- How often do the symptoms occur? Every day or night? Just a few times a week? Once a week or less?

- When do the symptoms happen? Does your child cough more at night and when she first wakes up in the morning?

Triggers: Next, the doctor will ask about things you may have noticed that make your child's symptoms worse. The list of possible asthma triggers is long, but it's very important to go through all of them to help pinpoint exactly what brings on your child's symptoms or makes them worse. The asthma triggers your doctor will ask about include:

- Colds, respiratory infections, sore throats, ear infections, sinus infections
- Allergens, such as mold, dust mites, furry or feathered animals, pollen
- Running, active play, exercise
- Tobacco smoke
- Cold weather or big changes in the weather
- Woodsmoke from a stove or fireplace
- Foods that contain additives and preservatives
- Certain medicines, such as aspirin

If being around any of the typical asthma triggers makes your child's symptoms worse, that is the clue that asthma is the problem. Knowing which triggers affect your child is an important part of asthma treatment. Discovering and treating your child's allergies, for instance, will do a lot to help her asthma. You can also take simple steps at home to reduce or eliminate her exposure to triggers. (More about this will be given in chapter 10.)

Severity: The next important step in understanding your child's symptom pattern is to gauge how severe symptoms are. Your doctor will want to know:

- Do the symptoms interfere with daily activities such as eating, walking, and playing quietly?
- Do the symptoms wake your child up in the night or keep her from napping?
- Do the symptoms keep your child home from school or daycare or keep your child from doing well in school?

- Have you called the doctor or brought your child to the doctor's office for unscheduled visits because of asthma symptoms?
- Has your child needed to go to the emergency room or been hospitalized because of asthma symptoms?
- What helps alleviate the wheezing, including any medicines?

Your doctor may have already prescribed a trial of an inhaled medicine to help open your child's breathing tubes even before a diagnosis of asthma is made. If so, you'll be asked if your child needs the medicine more often than before. All this information is important for helping the doctor understand the symptom pattern that points to asthma.

It can be very difficult for a parent to know or remember over a period of several weeks exactly what seems to make symptoms worse or how often or when they occur. You cannot always tell which triggers are around your child, because many allergens, such as pollen or dust mites, are invisible. To help you keep track of your child's symptoms, many doctors and nurse practitioners suggest keeping written notes over several weeks.

Being able to tell the doctor exactly how many times your child woke up in the night with wheezing and coughing, for instance, will be a big help in deciding whether asthma is the problem and how severe the asthma is. You're probably not around your child all the time, so ask other caregivers and your child herself (if she's old enough to understand) about asthma symptoms. Bring your notes with you to the doctor's office to help everyone get a better idea of your child's symptom pattern.

EXAMINING YOUR CHILD

After talking to you and your child about symptoms, the doctor will give your child a physical exam. The doctor will look at the child's nose, throat, and ears to check for secretions (runny nose), swollen mucous membranes, and infections. Rhinitis (runny nose), sinusitis (sinus infection), and ear infections can cause coughing similar to asthma—and they can also be asthma triggers. Nasal polyps (growths in the nose that block the sinuses) can sometimes be seen in children with allergies and asthma. The doctor will also look at the child's skin for signs of dermatitis or eczema, rashes often caused by allergies. Children with skin allergies are more prone to asthma.

If your child is feeling well—and even if he isn't—it's quite possible that the doctor won't hear any wheezing when listening to his chest with a stethoscope. This can be a little frustrating to a parent who has been hearing a child wheeze every morning for days. You might be afraid that the doctor won't believe you when you say your child wheezes or might think you're being overprotective. Don't worry. Experienced doctors know that asthma symptoms vary through the day. The child who wheezes at night or first thing in the morning may sound fine that afternoon in the office, but he will still wheeze again that night.

Wheezing is an important asthma symptom, but it's not the only one. In fact, many children with asthma never wheeze—coughing and shortness of breath are their main symptoms. If a child is actively wheezing, the doctor will look for other signs of labored breathing, such as retractions (a drawing-in of the skin between the ribs that indicates more vigorous "sucking in" of air), flaring of the nostrils, and/or bluish tint to the skin or nail beds, which indicates the child is not getting enough oxygen. You can check for these asthma signs at home as well.

BREATHING TESTS

Based on family medical history and your child's medical history and symptoms, the doctor may strongly suspect your child has asthma. The doctor may want your child to have other tests to be certain of the diagnosis and to determine how severe the asthma is and what treatment steps to take. One of these is a special breathing test known as pulmonary function testing (PFTs) or *spirometry*.

Spirometry measures how much the airways are blocked by the swelling and squeezing of asthma. The test is a bit complicated and needs some special equipment, but it's not at all painful and doesn't take very long. Not every physician has a spirometer machine in the office, so you may need to go to an asthma specialist or hospital clinic to have the test done.

To take this test, your child will sit up straight in a chair, breathe in as deeply as she can, and then breathe out as hard as she can into a special mouthpiece. To make sure that all the exhaled air goes into the mouthpiece, the doctor or respiratory therapist will gently pinch the child's nose closed with special soft clips. You can prepare your child for spirometry by explaining that it's very much like blowing out candles on a birthday cake.

The air goes from the mouthpiece through a tube and into a machine that measures how much air she breathed out, and how fast it came out. The measurements look at three things:

- FEV1, or *forced expiratory volume in one second*. This is the amount of air exhaled during the first second as a child breathes out hard. This measures the size of your child's airways.

- FVC, or *forced vital capacity*. This measures the size of your child's lungs.

- PEF, or *peak expiratory flow*. This measures how fast the air is exhaled when the child starts to breathe out. It is another indicator of airway size.

Your child will repeat the "maneuver," as this process is called, at least three times in a row to be sure the reading is accurate. Each maneuver only takes about six seconds. The results are compared to a table of typical results for your child's gender, age, ethnicity, and height. Your child's readings will be a percentage of normal based on the tables.

After the first round of maneuvers is over, the doctor may give your child a dose of an inhaled bronchodilator, a drug that opens up the breathing tubes. After giving the drug about fifteen to twenty minutes to work, your child will repeat the breathing maneuvers another three times. If your child has asthma, the results should be noticeably better this time because the bronchodilator will have opened the airways, allowing more air to move in and out. If that happens, the doctor will say that the airflow obstruction is reversible—in other words, medicines help reduce the bronchospasm/squeezing that blocks the airways. This is extremely important in determining that the problem is asthma.

By comparing the FEV1 before and after use of the bronchodilator, a physician can get a clear idea of the reversibility of the airway obstruction. This information helps the doctor decide which medicines are needed and what the starting doses should be.

Is this test necessary? Spirometry is a very good way to confirm that a child has asthma, even if a doctor is already quite certain. Spirometry is also important for helping a physician decide how severe the asthma is and what the best treatment would be. Once the treatment has started and your child's asthma has been under control for a few months, the doctor will want your child to repeat the test. This will help make sure the airways are as open and near normal as possible. After these initial tests, your child should have spirometry at least once a year simply to be sure the airways are staying at or near normal. If a child has a change in treatment—for example, a change in the dosage of her medicine— she may need spirometry again to be sure that the new treatment is working well.

If your child is younger than four or five, you're probably wondering how a spirometry maneuver can ever be done with a baby, a toddler, or even a preschooler. It can't. But doctors can do specialized breathing tests on babies and young children. These tests are more complex and require special equipment. If your doctor feels these tests are needed, you'll probably have to go to a specialist based at a large hospital.

Sometimes older children can't manage the spirometry maneuver either. When a child can't do it for some reason, doctors may suggest a "therapeutic trial," which means trying an inhaled bronchodilator or steroid pills for a short time. (These medicines will be discussed in detail in chapter 5.) Seeing if one of these medicines helps reduce wheezing and other symptoms is a way to help determine whether the child has asthma.

Some children have asthma symptoms, but their spirometry results are normal. In that case, a doctor may recommend a different type of spirometry test called bronchoprovocation. In this test, a child inhales a small, safe amount of a substance called methacholine. If the child has asthma, the methacholine will make her airways constrict or squeeze just as if she were having mild asthma symptoms. When she does the spirometry maneuvers after taking the medicine, her readings will be lower. If she doesn't have asthma, the methacholine will have little effect, and the spirometry readings will be nearly the same as before. A similar test can be done using another medication called histamine. In a third test, a child breathes cold dry air or gets on a bicycle or treadmill and does vigorous exercise. All of these tests may cause bronchoconstriction in children with asthma and are useful in confirming the diagnosis.

Other tests, such as a chest X-ray, a sweat test, barium swallow exam, or allergy testing, may be done to help rule out other causes of the symptoms or to identify factors that might complicate your child's asthma.

HOW BAD IS IT?

Based on symptoms, physical examination, and the results of spirometry, the physician will determine the severity of your child's asthma. Severity falls into four basic classifications, or steps:

- **Step 1, mild intermittent:** Symptoms occur during the day or night no more than two days a week or two nights a month. Flare-ups of symptoms are short, and often there are no symptoms between flares. The child's FEV1 is 80 percent or more of normal.

- **Step 2, mild persistent:** Symptoms occur two or more times a week but less than daily; nighttime symptoms occur more than two times a month. Physical activity levels are affected by flares. The child's FEV1 is still 80 percent or more of normal.

- **Step 3, moderate persistent:** Symptoms occur every day; nighttime symptoms occur once a week or more. Physical activity levels are affected by flares. The child's FEV1 is 60 to 80 percent of normal.

- **Step 4, severe persistent:** Symptoms occur continuously, with frequent flares; symptoms occur frequently at night. Physical activity is decreased. The child's FEV1 is 60 percent or less of normal.

It's very important to remember that asthma severity can change. Any child with asthma may step up or down to a different level at any time. The symptoms may get better, or they may get suddenly worse. Children with asthma, no matter what their classification, can have severe asthma flares. Everyone responsible for your child needs to be alert for changes in your child's asthma and aware that flares can happen unexpectedly.

Specialist Care

Does your child need to see an asthma specialist? This depends on severity. If your child's asthma is at Step 3 or higher and requires daily preventative medicine, or if your child is under five years old, it is probably a good idea to work with a specialist, especially when designing the original treatment plan. It may be useful for children whose asthma is at Step 2 to see an asthma specialist as well; for instance, if their symptoms are not responding to the treatment plan or for advice about whether treatment should be changed. Pediatricians who specialize in asthma are usually pediatric pulmonologists (lung specialists) or pediatric allergists (allergy specialists). They have had advanced training and are highly experienced in treating asthma. Studies have shown that children who see asthma specialists are less likely to end up in the emergency room and hospital with severe flares. Asthma specialists are very familiar with the best practice guidelines for treating asthma and with the latest research.

If your pediatrician suspects your child has asthma, you may be referred to a specialist right away, especially if the asthma is severe, if the doctor can't do spirometry in the office, or if the child is under age three. There are several other good reasons to see a specialist as part of diagnosing asthma:

- The child has had a life-threatening asthma flare.
- The child has other health problems, such as rhinitis or sinusitis, that make the asthma worse.

- The child needs to be tested or treated for allergies.
- The child has breathing problems but doesn't have typical asthma symptoms.
- The child is taking asthma medicines but isn't getting better.
- There is concern that the symptoms may be caused by an illness other than asthma.

Once asthma has been diagnosed and its severity determined, developing a treatment approach is the next step. You the parent, the specialist, and the pediatrician will need to decide how to manage the treatment. For mild cases (Step 1 and Step 2) in older children, a pediatrician may be the best and most convenient doctor to follow your child. But asthma unfortunately doesn't always stay at the milder steps. If the treatment doesn't seem to be helping, if your child is still having flares, or if she needs to take a lot of oral steroids or use high doses of inhaled steroids to treat symptoms, it's definitely time to see the specialist again. With the right treatment, even severe, persistent asthma can be controlled. Insist on nothing less for your child.

3

The Asthma-Allergy Connection

The link between allergies and asthma is very strong. Most children with asthma—probably as many as 80 percent—have allergies, and 40 percent of children with allergies in the nose (hay fever or allergic rhinitis, for example) also have asthma symptoms.

The key point is this: if you can control children's allergies, their asthma symptoms will be less intense and less frequent. To understand and manage asthma successfully, it's important to know something about allergies.

HOW DO ALLERGIES OCCUR?

Allergies are a common problem that affects at least two of every ten Americans. Simply put, people with allergies react to certain substances called *allergens*—dust, pollen, animal dander, mold, or smoke, for example—that don't cause reactions in other people. An allergic person's immune system responds to allergens like a false alarm. When an allergen triggers the immune system—setting off the alarm—the body reacts by sneezing, wheezing, coughing, and/or itching, depending on what particular part of the body has the reaction. Other allergens in foods cause a skin or intestinal reaction.

A quick biology lesson: our bodies make immunoglobulins to help fight various infections. There are five different types of immunoglobulin: IgG, IgA, IgM, IgE, and IgD. IgG, IgA, and IgM are some of the body's most important weapons against bacterial infections. The allergic antibody called IgE (immunoglobulin E) is part of the body's natural response for fighting other types of infections, particularly parasites like worms. In someone with allergies, the body recognizes certain allergens as foreign invaders and makes more IgE. Everyone makes some IgE, but allergic children make more IgE in reaction to pollen and dust than a nonallergic child does.

An allergic reaction starts when an allergen attaches to the allergen-specific-IgE antibody and activates certain cells, including "mast cells" found in skin and tissues that line the nose, throat, and lungs. An IgE antibody that attaches to a mast cell acts like a fuse on a bomb. When IgE antibody's specific allergen comes along, it's like touching a match to the fuse—the antibody makes the mast cell burst open and release a number of substances, including one called histamine that causes redness, swelling, and itching.

Location is everything. The site where histamine is released determines the type of reaction. When histamine is released in the tissues lining the nose, the results are redness, itching, swelling, sneezing, and a runny nose—what allergists call allergic rhinitis, but most people simply call it hay fever. (In this chapter, the two terms will be used interchangeably.) When histamine is released in the skin, the results are itching, rashes, and hives causing atopic dermatitis, or eczema. When histamine is released in the stomach, it causes cramping and diarrhea. When histamine is released in the lungs, it causes airways to tighten, swell up, and produce extra mucus—the recipe for asthma.

To develop an allergy, a child needs to be exposed to the allergen several times. The first few exposures cause the immune system to make more IgE. Subsequent exposures will cause the body to respond to the IgE and allergen by releasing histamine, and then symptoms will appear.

This is why many children do not have allergy symptoms in the first few years of life but develop them during their school-age years or later.

ARE ALLERGIES INHERITED?

Although there are many reasons why allergies are so common, family history is by far the most important. The genetic tendency to have allergies, called *atopy*, is inherited. If one parent has allergies, a child has a fifty-fifty chance of having allergies. If both parents have allergies, a child has about a 70 percent chance of developing allergies. You might assume that if you are allergic only to a certain tree pollen, for example, your child will react to the same allergen, but that's not always the case. Your daughter could be allergic to dogs and your son to molds. The tendency to have allergies is inherited, but *the specific allergy isn't* because children don't always share the same allergies with their parents.

ARE ALLERGIES BECOMING MORE WIDESPREAD?

Yes, allergies are increasing. We do not know why the incidence rates of allergies are rising, but they are. Asthma, hay fever, eczema, and food allergies are all on the increase. The most common theory to explain the rising numbers is the hygiene theory. This theory is based on the belief that young people today are cleaner and come in contact with fewer germs than previous generations. This doesn't mean that we clean our homes more often or more thoroughly today. It means that we are exposed to fewer bacterial products because of an increased use of antibiotics; it also means that more people are living in cities and suburbs instead of working on farms where they have greater exposure to animal bacteria. Unfortunately, this doesn't account for all the increases in allergies. People who work on farms or with farm animals still develop allergies.

Some of the increased incidence of allergies may be attributed simply to the fact that we have improved diagnosis and a better count of allergy sufferers than ever before. As public awareness about allergies has grown, people seek diagnosis and treatment, so we have a more accurate picture of how many individuals really have allergies. But even taking into account this increased diagnosis, allergies are on the rise worldwide.

THE ATOPIC TRIAD

Allergy symptoms vary, depending on what parts of the body are affected. Many children have allergies in three areas—the skin, lungs, and nose. When this occurs, it is called the atopic triad. But allergies in children tend to move from one area of the body to another. About 10 to 15 percent of all youngsters develop allergies in their skin (atopic dermatitis, also called eczema) during infancy and early childhood. Atopic dermatitis is a very itchy red rash that comes and goes. Many children outgrow this allergy by age five to eight, only later to develop hay fever or other allergies in their noses. About half of all children with atopic dermatitis also develop asthma.

Allergic rhinitis can affect as many as 40 percent of all children at some point in their lives. Although the name hay fever suggests that it occurs only during the "allergy season" of spring and fall, many children have symptoms year-round. That's because allergic rhinitis is caused not only by plant pollen but also by many other allergens that are ever present in the air, such as mold spores, animal dander, and dust.

Allergic rhinitis is a major reason for missed school days. Symptoms alone can be severe enough to keep a child home, but children with allergic rhinitis are also more likely to develop other problems, including ear infections (otitis media), inflamed sinuses around the nose (sinusitis), red, watery, itchy eyes (allergic conjunctivitis), as well as asthma.

Allergic rhinitis and asthma go hand in hand because both are inflammatory diseases with the same underlying cause. Because the linings of the upper airways—the nose, sinuses, mouth, and throat—are connected to the linings of the airways in the lungs, they are affected by the same things and respond in similar ways.

Almost 80 percent of children with asthma also have allergic rhinitis, and close to 40 percent of those with allergic rhinitis also have asthma. So it's clear that treating allergic rhinitis to reduce the swelling in the nose and upper airways can help reduce swelling in the lower airways. By using proper medicine to treat allergic rhinitis and by avoiding allergens whenever possible, children can have fewer asthma symptoms and flares.

COMMON ALLERGENS

Allergens typically include dust mites, animal dander, pollens, and molds. Here is a brief description of the usual suspects:

Dust Mites

Probably the most common allergens of all, dust mites are microscopic creatures related to spiders. They live by the millions in every home—in mattresses, pillows, bedding, cushions, upholstery, carpets, stuffed animals, draperies, clothing, towels, and just about anywhere else, especially where dust accumulates. They feed on the tiny particles of dead skin that humans and animals constantly shed. Dust mite droppings and the body parts of dead dust mites float in the air—in fact, they make up a good part of house dust. The droppings and particles are very, very allergenic.

Dust mites are not an indictment of your housekeeping skills—they're just a fact of life. You can never get rid of them completely, but you can reduce your child's exposure quite a bit by encasing her mattress and pillow in a special hypoallergenic cover, washing bedding and stuffed toys in hot water (120°F), having a two-ply bag or HEPA filter for your vacuum cleaner, removing carpets and rugs where possible, and keeping the humidity in the house between 30 and 50 percent. Dust mites like to grow in moderate temperatures and high humidity, so taking the above measures can reduce dust mite levels by 100 to 1,000-fold.

Pollen

Most people recognize pollen as that fine-grained, greenish yellow powder that dusts windowsills and cars parked under trees in the spring. But there are many types of pollens, seen and unseen. Pollens are tiny male cells of flowering plants that fertilize female plant cells so seeds can form. These plant pollens are most likely to cause allergies. They rely on the wind for fertilization and are generally very fine, dry, and light, so they get into the air easily.

Pollen can travel hundreds of miles, so you do not have to live near its source to have symptoms. When eight-year-old Billy started sneezing and wheezing, his parents didn't suspect a pollen allergy, for example, because they lived on the fifteenth floor of an apartment building, high above the trees and twelve blocks from the nearest park, in the middle of the city. Yet pollen turned out to be the villain that triggered Billy's reaction.

Pollen season depends on where you live. The two main seasons, spring and fall, vary according to local climate, trees, grasses, and shrubs. Pollen appears during the growing seasons of trees and grasses. In the South, grass pollen season lasts longer than grass season in the North. Tree pollen develops just as leaves start to sprout. In the North, early spring marks the beginning of pollen season, while it may start earlier or extend later in the South. The amount of pollen produced also depends on local vegetation. For example, ragweed grows most prolifically in the Midwest and Northeast, so these regions have the highest ragweed pollen levels.

Pollen counts can also change over time in various areas of the country. In fact, the deserts of the Southwest used to be fairly pollen-free, but they now have a rampant pollen problem because many people moved there from other, greener parts of the country and planted trees, grasses, and shrubs that are thriving in the warm climate and giving off tons of pollen.

Pollen counts are generally classified as low, moderate, high, and very high. If the counts are low, only individuals who are extremely sensitive to these pollens and molds will experience symptoms. If the counts are moderate, many people will have symptoms. If the counts are high, most individuals will show symptoms, and if the counts are very high, almost everyone with any sensitivity at all to these pollens and molds will experience symptoms.

The following table shows pollen count classifications. Keep in mind, however, that pollen counts reported by TV, radio, Web sites, and newspapers usually lag a day or two behind the current day's count.

Pollen Count Classifications

	Grass	Molds	Trees	Weeds
Absent	0	0	0	0
Low	1–4	1–6,499	1–14	1–9
Moderate	5–9	6,500–12,999	15–89	10–49
High	10–199	13,000–49,999	90–1,499	50–499
Very High	>200	>50,000	>1,500	>500

The allergy season depends largely on weather conditions as well as location, but pollen problems in general start in February or March and run through October. The only real break from pollen comes in cold winter weather. As a general rule, allergies will be better—less bothersome—on rainy or windless days and worse when the weather is hot, dry, or windy.

It is difficult to avoid airborne pollens, but some simple tricks do help. To bring fresh air into a room in the spring and fall, use an air conditioner instead of a window fan because the air conditioner will filter out most pollen particles. Children should wash their hands and faces when they come in from outside and bathe before bedtime to remove pollen from their skin. And one other tip: laundry should not be dried outdoors where it can accumulate pollen.

Molds

Molds are microscopic fungi that reproduce by spores, not by pollen or seeds. Like pollen, mold spores are extremely small and light so they are easily carried by air currents. Unlike pollen, however, mold spores are found just about everywhere, both indoors and outdoors, and are present year-round. The easiest way to avoid indoor molds is to *decrease the humidity* level of the house to less than 50 percent. Do not use a humidifier in the winter. Using bleach to clean bathrooms, kitchens, and air vents and filters also helps reduce mold exposure.

Mold spores are present outdoors throughout the year in soil, vegetation, dead leaves, and similar environments. In temperate areas, mold spores tend to peak outdoors from March to October, but in warmer areas mold spores are around all the time. Indoors, mold spores in the form of mildew and other types of fungus are found year-round in attics, basements, bathrooms, refrigerators, carpets, upholstery, and just about anyplace, especially where it's damp and dark.

When considering how to reduce your child's exposure to pollen and molds, remember: the more pollens and mold spores are carried by air currents, the worse allergy symptoms will be.

Animal Dander

All furry or feathered animals constantly shed particles—hair, bits of feather, tiny skin flakes called dander, and drops of saliva—that trigger allergies. Though it's difficult for many pet lovers to accept, *there are no nonallergic dogs and cats.* All dogs and cats have dander and saliva that can cause problems for a child who is sensitive to these allergens. The only way to control animal dander is to remove the animal from the environment. Unfortunately, it takes six to twelve months after the animal leaves the home for dander levels to be reduced to a nonallergenic point.

For some families, it is impossible to remove a pet from the home. In these cases, the pet should not go into the child's bedroom or in a car with the child. Washing the pet weekly also can reduce the level of dander.

Recent studies have examined the role of pets in allergies and asthma. It is clear that if a child is allergic to pets, having a pet at home will make the asthma or allergies worse. Interestingly, however, if parents already have a pet in the home before a child is born or when the child is an infant, their child may be less likely to develop allergies to pets. Exact recommendations for whether or not to keep a pet in your home and whether or not the pet is making your child's asthma and allergies worse depends on each individual child. The decision to keep a pet or not should be discussed with your doctor or nurse practitioner.

Cockroaches

The cockroach connection to allergies and asthma is very strong. Cockroaches are the major allergen for children who live in cities. Many children are highly sensitive to cockroach saliva, droppings, and body parts, which are so light that they float in the air as part of house dust. No matter how well you clean your home, cockroaches are found everywhere. But they are especially a problem in older housing and multifamily dwellings. Cockroaches themselves and cockroach allergens can be difficult to control. The best controls include professional extermination, keeping the kitchen clean, storing food in sealed containers, keeping the house (especially bathrooms and basements) dry, using cockroach traps, and sealing cracks in walls and floors.

REDUCING ALLERGENS

Environmental controls—removing or reducing allergens around your child—can make a significant difference to your child's health. You may not be able to eliminate every single trace of allergens, but the more you reduce exposure to the things you know cause problems, the happier and healthier your child will be.

Children don't have to live in a bubble and parents don't have to become crazed super-housekeepers to do this. You can't avoid all allergens all the time, but many simple, commonsense steps can reduce environmental allergens and other asthma triggers quickly and easily. (More information about these steps will be given in chapter 10.) For now, think of your child's allergies as a bucket. Over the course of a day, each allergen she encounters fills the bucket a little more until finally it overflows and allergy or asthma symptoms flare. You may not be able to keep the allergy bucket from filling up a little, but you can definitely take steps that will help keep it from spilling over.

FOOD ALLERGIES

Occasionally children with asthma also have food allergies that can cause wheezing. It is very rare, however, that asthma is the only symptom of food allergies. Most children with a food allergy react with hives, rash, vomiting, diarrhea, and/or wheezing. Foods that most often cause allergies are eggs, milk, wheat, nuts, peanuts, and soy. Children with allergies to eggs are more likely to have asthma than all other children. Often—but not always—children outgrow allergies to milk, egg, soy, and wheat by the time they are four or five years old.

If you suspect your child has food allergies, it is extremely important to find out exactly which foods are the problem and avoid them completely. Food allergies can cause very severe, even life-threatening reactions. Though you may have heard otherwise, food dyes and preservatives do not cause food allergies or asthma symptoms.

IDENTIFYING ALLERGIES

How can you tell if your child has allergies? After your child has been diagnosed with asthma, your physician or nurse practitioner may recommend allergy testing. If a tendency toward allergies runs in your family, allergy testing is even more important. By identifying and treating your child's allergies, you'll be doing a lot to reduce his asthma symptoms as well.

As with asthma itself, the first step in diagnosing allergies is a detailed family history and a discussion of your child's symptom pattern. Knowing the type and pattern of symptoms is most helpful when making a diagnosis. For example, Charlotte's parents noticed this pattern and reported it to her doctor: Charlotte sneezes most often in the fall (even though she doesn't have a head cold) and when she's around the neighbor's dog. She is probably allergic to ragweed and animals. After the history is reviewed, the doctor will examine Charlotte and look for specific allergy symptoms.

The following descriptions can help you identify symptoms and patterns that you can relay to your child's doctor and will be useful in diagnosis and treatment:

The intensely itchy rash of atopic dermatitis is usually easy to spot. In babies and young children, the rash is often on the face and scalp, but it may appear just about anywhere on the body except the diaper area. In older children, the rash is usually found where the skin creases at the elbows, knees, and neck, although it can also appear on the wrists, hands, ankles, and feet as well.

You may have noticed the most obvious symptoms of allergic rhinitis including:

- Sneezing many times in a row
- Clear discharge from a continuously runny nose
- Itchy nose, ears, mouth
- Red, itchy eyes
- "Allergic shiners," those black circles under a child's eyes caused by nasal congestion
- The allergic salute: the child frequently swipes his hand upward across the tip of his nose

As a side effect of the clogged nasal passages caused by allergic rhinitis, a child may have frequent ear infections or sinusitis that, in turn, can cause asthma flares. When the swelling from allergic rhinitis blocks a child's ears, she can't hear as well as usual. Allergic rhinitis may also make her irritable and tired, and it could affect her ability to concentrate in school.

ALLERGY TESTING

A doctor needs to know exactly what your child is allergic to in order to treat allergies effectively. The best way to detect particular allergies is by taking a type of skin test called a prick or scratch test. Skin testing is the quickest and easiest way to test a child's reaction to a large number of allergens all at once. By using this technique a doctor will be able to give you an answer usually within fifteen minutes.

To do a skin test, a doctor or nurse will place small drop of each different allergen on the arm or back. The drop is then scratched with a special fork or needle. Sometimes the drop and scratch are done at the same time. If a child is allergic to a certain substance, the skin of that scratch will react by swelling and turning red, usually within fifteen minutes or so. The reaction dies down again quickly, usually within another thirty minutes.

Skin testing may sound painful, but it hardly hurts at all. The special forks or needles that the doctor uses are very fine and barely penetrate the top layer of skin. The swelling from any reactions goes away quickly, although the area may feel itchy for a few hours. You can prepare your child for skin testing by explaining the procedure in advance and assuring him that the scratches will be shallow, the needles will be very thin, and it won't hurt. In fact, it's nothing like getting a shot.

Skin testing can be done safely on children of any age, even infants. If your child has been taking any antihistamines (medications to treat allergy symptoms), it's important for him to stop taking them before the test or the results won't be accurate. If your child takes antihistamines or any other medicines, discuss them with the doctor well in advance of the testing. Your child may have to stop taking the medication temporarily.

Dangerous reactions to skin testing are very rare, but they are possible, so the test must be done by a specialist in a medical office where the equipment and staff are available to treat a bad reaction. If the itching from the skin tests doesn't go away after a few hours, or if a child is short of breath or wheezes after the test, he could be having a bad reaction to the skin testing. Call the doctor at once or go to the nearest emergency room.

Skin testing is a highly reliable way to identify allergies, but it's not always completely accurate. Sometimes a child can have a strong allergic reaction to something but have a negative skin test for the same substance. Because there are many possible reasons for this, your allergist will probably want to do other tests.

If results of the scratch test are unclear, in some cases the allergist will inject a tiny amount of an allergen directly under the skin, usually on the upper arm, to see if there is a reaction. This sort of skin testing is a bit more uncomfortable, but the needle is hardly noticeable and the reaction, if there is one, is very mild.

Another type of allergy testing is called *radioallergosorbent blood test*, or RAST for short. This test uses a blood sample to check for different IgE antibodies. It's more expensive than skin testing, and the results can take as long as two weeks to become available. RAST testing is generally used only when skin testing can't be done—for instance, if the child has extensive eczema, has to take a medicine every day, or has asthma that isn't under control.

With all these tests, a false negative result may occur, which means allergic symptoms are evident, but the test is negative. The test results, therefore, have to be interpreted along with the history and physical exam that your physician had done previously.

TREATING ALLERGIES

The most effective and inexpensive way to treat allergies is to avoid all allergens whenever possible, but it's easier to avoid some than others. You can reduce your child's exposure to certain allergens—like keeping him away from smoke or pets if those trigger his allergies. But your child cannot and should not stay indoors all the time, so outdoor pollens cannot be avoided entirely.

The alternative to avoiding allergens is to use various medicines to control allergy symptoms. The best medicines are those used directly on the site of symptoms: nasal sprays for hay fever and ointments and creams for the skin for atopic dermatitis.

Nasal Sprays

For children with allergic rhinitis, doctors generally prefer to prescribe nasal corticosteroid sprays to help relieve symptoms. These medicines are the most effective because they block the cells that cause symptoms instead of treating each symptom individually. These drugs, including beclomethasone (Beconase), budesonide (Rhinocort), mometasone (Nasonex), triamcilone (Nasalcort), and fluticasone (Flonase), are very effective and very safe. These medicines have been approved for various ages (some for children as young as three) and are usually used once a day. The most common side effect is a nosebleed, which can be controlled when nasal sprays are used correctly. The corticosteroid nasal spray should be sprayed into the nose with the tip of the spray pointed up and outward toward the eye or about 45 degrees away from the center of the nose.

Cromolyn nose spray (Nasalcrom) is an alternative to corticosteroid sprays. Cromolyn is very safe but less effective than nasal corticosteroids. Cromolyn is available in nonprescription form, but talk to your child's doctor before using it to be sure this is the best treatment for your child.

Medicines for the Skin

The most effective treatment for atopic dermatitis is good skin care. Most children do better with a daily bath, frequent use of moisturizers, and use of mild, nondrying soaps. To control skin inflammation, redness, and itching, prescription medicines may be used. There are two types of topical medicines. ("Topical" just means it is applied directly to the skin.) They are corticosteroids and macrolides, a nonsteroid medicine. Topical corticosteroids range in strength from mild to very potent. Low potency topical steroids like hydrocortisone do not have the side effects seen in high potency topical steroids. The more potent ones can cause thinned skin, stretch marks, and other problems if used too many days in the same area of the body. To prevent side effects, your doctor may limit the length of treatment time and locations where these ointments should be applied.

The macrolides are fairly new topical medicines and have been approved for use since February 2000. Tacrolimus (Protopic) and pimecrolimus (Elidel) are two examples of this new class of medicine that inhibits the activity of cells that play a role in eczema. Studies have shown that this new class of drugs will improve or completely clear eczema in 60 to 80 percent of treated patients. The major side effect seen in these medicines is some itching or burning in the first week of use.

Antihistamines

The most popular medicines for allergies are antihistamines. As the name suggests, antihistamines counteract the swelling and other effects of histamine. They are very effective for keeping allergy symptoms from starting and for treating them when they do.

The most widely used antihistamines today are called H_1 receptor antagonists and are available by prescription only. They are sometimes also called second-generation antihistamines because they have taken over from the older, first-generation antihistamines that used to cause drowsiness. H_1 receptor antagonists block the release of histamine and help reduce or prevent inflammation. They dry up runny noses, stop sneezing, and help prevent wheezing. Desloratadine (Clarinex), fexofenadine (Allegra), and cetirizine (Zyrtec) are the most commonly prescribed antihistamines and have been approved for children as young as two years of age. They're also long-lasting, and some are available in syrups or dissolving tablets to make dosing easier for young children. Your doctor will choose which medication to prescribe, depending on your child's age and symptoms.

In 2002, a formerly prescribed H_1 receptor antagonist antihistamine, loratadine (Claritin), became available as an over-the-counter medicine (OTC, or nonprescription). OTC antihistamines such as Actifed, Benadryl, or Tavist can relieve allergy symptoms but will probably make your child drowsy. It is best, therefore, to talk to a doctor before giving any OTC medicines to your child.

Decongestants

Decongestants are sometimes used in addition to nasal sprays and antihistamines to reduce the congestion that some people have with allergic rhinitis. Nonprescription decongestants in pill or syrup form are sold separately and are also found in many nonprescription allergy formulas along with an antihistamine. These medicines usually contain a drug called pseudoephedrine that can make your child irritable or hyperactive. Talk to your doctor before using any of these products. Oral nonprescription spray decongestants, such as phenylephrine (Neo-Synephrine), are safe for occasional use but shouldn't be used for more than a day or two. If they are used longer, your child's body could react with rebound congestion, which is stuffiness and/or a runny nose that are made even worse by overuse of the decongestant.

Allergy Shots

The final step in treating a child's allergies is allergen immunotherapy, better known as allergy shots. These shots work by repeatedly giving a child a very small, controlled dose of the allergens that affect him. Allergen immunotherapy eventually slows or even stops his reaction. Think of it as training the child's immune system to stop interpreting an allergen as a threat.

Allergy immunotherapy is highly effective and usually reduces symptoms and the number of medicines that children need to control their symptoms of allergies and asthma. The most exciting potential benefit is that it might prevent additional allergies from developing. Children who might benefit from allergy shots:

- Have allergies all or most of the year
- Are allergic to things that can't be avoided, such as pollen
- Need to take a lot of medicines to control allergy symptoms
- Need to take medicine to treat another ongoing health problem, and those medicines are affected by allergy medicines
- Do not respond to or do not tolerate medicines
- Cannot use or are unwilling to use medicines

Allergy shots are not for everyone. They may have side effects because they give a child the very allergen that she is allergic to. Side effects or reactions tend to occur in the first thirty minutes after the shot. The most common side effect is a hive or rash at the site of injection.

Other more serious side effects include coughing, wheezing, or anaphylaxis (the whole body reacts). Allergy shots, therefore, should only be given in a doctor's office, and a thirty-minute wait is recommended before leaving the office.

Another problem with immunotherapy is that it takes a long time to work. A child will need to get shots at the doctor's office once or twice a week for about six months. With each shot, the amount of the allergen is increased a bit. After about four to six months, the amount of the allergen reaches a steady, even level. Called the maintenance dose, it is given each week and slowly extended to every three or four weeks for the next three to five years.

Whatever allergy treatments you and your child's doctor decide to pursue, remember this basic fact: keeping the allergy symptoms at bay will go a long way toward keeping your child's asthma under good control.

4

Taking Control of Asthma

The most effective way to manage a chronic condition like asthma is to keep it *under control*. We know that there is no cure for asthma, so the very best we can do as parents and health care professionals is to control it by preventing airway inflammation and minimizing triggers that can set off a flare.

When asthma is described as a *chronic* condition or illness, it means that it is ongoing, month to month, year to year. This doesn't mean that asthma symptoms stay at a steady level of frequency or intensity. A key to understanding any chronic disease is recognizing that it *changes* over time. Chronic illnesses—for example, asthma, diabetes, inflammatory bowel disease, cystic fibrosis—behave like seesaws. There are ups and downs, good times when symptoms are quiet or even nonexistent, and other times when they become aggressive.

This uneven course often confuses parents and children alike because it's difficult to understand and accept asthma's changes. Sometimes your child may have many frequent symptoms that require a lot of medicine (maybe more than you feel comfortable giving your child). At other times when you observe no symptoms, it may seem that your child needs no medicine at all.

How will you know if your child's asthma is under the best control possible? Or when it's fairly well controlled but not as much as it could be? Making these assessments isn't easy or clear-cut. There's no red warning light that's either on or off. No alarm bells will ring to let you know that control is slipping. But you don't have to grope in the dark either. There are guidelines for determining the degree of asthma control, even as the disease takes its typical waxing and waning course.

A panel of asthma experts at the National Institutes of Health reviewed all the research available about asthma and used this information to set standards for asthma care. The panel developed guidelines to inform health care providers about diagnosing asthma, deciding how severe it is, treating it, and educating patients and families about asthma. In fact, these national guidelines spell out exactly how to tell whether or not asthma is under control. Much of this chapter is based on those national guidelines.

Ask about these NIH guidelines the next time you go for a medical visit. It is important to work closely with health care professionals to determine whether or not your child's asthma is under control. If it is not, why? What needs to be done? You and your child's physician or nurse practitioner should discuss and come to an agreement about how to work toward achieving control; or if your child's asthma is already under control, then how to maintain it.

WHAT DOES "UNDER CONTROL" MEAN?

Three basic considerations help to determine how well controlled your child's asthma is at any time during the course of the disease. *If your child's asthma is under control, he or she should:*

- **Not be bothered** *day or night* **by symptoms,** such as coughing, wheezing, shortness of breath, or chest tightness. But remember, even when a child does not show symptoms, it doesn't mean the asthma has disappeared. A child can't always feel when his breathing tubes are inflamed. You can't see it in your child, but some degree of airway inflammation is always there.

- **Be able to take part in all normal activities,** such as lugging hefty bookbags, going up and down stairs, taking gym class, and playing sports. If your child gets tired or can't keep up with other youngsters his own age, something is wrong and his asthma is not under control.

  Certainly some children just don't like sports or have little talent for them, but all young people need regular exercise to be healthy, grow, and develop normally. When children stay away from physical activities, it may seem that they just aren't interested, but this can be a mistaken interpretation. Younger children especially may appear disinterested, but they simply can't (or won't) tell you that they aren't feeling up to par. Once these children get proper asthma treatment, they are able to enjoy playing. A result of bringing their asthma under control is that they become more physically active. (More about asthma, exercise, and sports will be given in chapter 11.)

- **Be able to get a good night's sleep.** If children wake up because they're bothered by symptoms or need to take medicine in the middle of the night, their asthma is not under control as much as it could be. If symptoms disturb them at night, they will not be well rested the next day and will either miss school completely or be less attentive in class. Uncontrolled asthma may not only cause children to miss a lot of school, but it can also affect your work schedule. If you are waking up at night to give medicine or check on your child's breathing, you may be late or absent from work the next day.

HOW TO TAKE CONTROL

When most people think about controlling a disease, the first thing that comes to mind is medicine. The next two chapters will discuss the full range of asthma medicines and how to use them. But for our purposes here, in discussing how to keep asthma under control, keep these few facts in mind:

- Asthma medicines fall into two categories: long-term controller medicines and quick-relief medicines. Most, but not all, controller medicines treat airway inflammation.

- There are two ways to control airway inflammation. One is to make the airways less irritated so that they're less likely to overreact and cause symptoms. Airway irritation can be reduced by taking anti-inflammatory controller medicines properly.
- The second strategy for controlling airway inflammation is to stay away from triggers that cause symptoms or make asthma worse. Sometimes it's easy to detect exactly which triggers irritate the airways and spark symptoms. At other times these triggers are more difficult to pinpoint.

Let's look at the issue of secondhand smoke exposure, for example. Secondhand smoke is an irritant that bothers everyone's lungs, including the smoker and anyone else who's exposed to the smoke, whether or not they have asthma. When a child with asthma lives in a home with a smoker, the smoker may be fooled into believing that the smoke doesn't bother the child because he doesn't cough or wheeze when the adult is smoking. As an irritant, however, the smoke may increase the level of airway inflammation that the child can't feel. But this doesn't mean that the smoke is not causing a problem. If we observe how children react, once the smoker at least goes outside or quits smoking, we find that their asthma comes under better control and they may need less medicine.

WHAT'S *NOT* NORMAL?

Adam is teenager who manages his asthma quite well most of the year. But he seems to have the most problems in the fall, usually during the last week in September around his birthday. Just about every September, Adam "celebrates" his birthday in the hospital. He and his family have come to accept this annual ritual as routine.

Some people with asthma believe that being treated in the emergency room or being hospitalized is a normal part of having asthma. But it shouldn't be so. If a child comes to the emergency room or is hospitalized, his asthma is not under control.

If your child's asthma gets out of control and he starts to have symptoms, it is important to think about what's going on. Can you identify what has triggered your child's symptoms? Once you have identified the trigger, you will need to work out a way to make sure your child stays away from that trigger as much as possible. And when those triggers do set off an asthma attack, you'll need a plan to bring it under control. (See pages 220–222 about asthma management plans and chapter 9 about asthma emergencies.)

LUNG FUNCTION

A breathing test called *spirometry* monitors lung function, or how well children breathe. To take this test, they breathe into a machine that may be hooked up to a computer that prints a report of the results in numbers and on a graph. According to the NIH guidelines, the tests should be repeated several times: first, when a child is diagnosed with asthma; after starting medicine to see how well it's working; and again at least every one to two years. The test is also recommended when a child has persistent wheezing.

Spirometry is recommended for anyone who has asthma. But because the test requires a fair degree of coordination and cooperation, not every child can successfully perform the test. Children under age four or five, as well as some older children, are not capable of performing the test voluntarily. Many primary care physicians and all specialists or hospitals have equipment and personnel that are needed to perform spirometry. With children over twelve years of age, this testing is straightforward and similar to adult testing. With younger children, health care workers who are experienced in obtaining good spirometry results from a young age group should perform the test.

Spirometry is a very useful tool for determining whether or not a child's asthma is under control. She may act and feel fine and have no symptoms, but if her spirometry results are below normal for a child of the same sex and size, or if previous testing has shown better results, then something is going on. Her asthma is not under control.

If your child's test results are below normal, it is crucial to discuss the results with your child's doctor or nurse practitioner to find out why and figure out what needs to be done to bring the asthma under control again. When a child's asthma is under control, the spirometry results should be normal or even above normal for that individual child.

BOTHERSOME SIDE EFFECTS

All medicines (including those that require a prescription, over-the-counter medicines, and herbs/nutritional supplements) can cause side effects. Each time a new medicine is prescribed for your child, you should be aware of possible side effects. But the NIH guidelines suggest that children undergoing asthma treatments should be able to tolerate all their medicines with minimal or no side effects.

Doctors or nurse practitioners should talk with you about what to do if any side effects do occur. If they don't bring up the subject, ask about potential side effects. Sometimes parents don't ask but only read the package insert. When you read about possible symptoms or problems in an insert, you may be overwhelmed, but the Food and Drug Administration (FDA) requires that *all* possible side effects must be included in that insert—even those that are extremely rare. Keep in mind that some side effects can be harmful, but many are harmless and just bothersome. It's best to discuss possible side effects directly with a physician or nurse before your child begins taking the medicine.

If your child does experience a troubling side effect—whether she takes a medicine every day or just for quick relief—it is very possible that the medicine isn't being used properly. Again, check this out with your physician or nurse practitioner. Children who don't take medicines at the right time and in the correct way won't be able to meet the goal of keeping asthma under control. It is essential to let your child's pediatrician or nurse practitioner know that she is experiencing a side effect. They will help you determine if it was a significant side effect and what should be done about it. Many asthma medicines are currently on the market, so if one causes a problem, the doctor may substitute another.

Do not stop a medicine suddenly without notifying your doctor.

Michael and his family learned this lesson the hard way. Michael started a new medicine to control his airway inflammation, but he broke out in a rash. His mother decided to stop the new medicine but didn't inform the pediatrician. The following week, Michael started wheezing during exercise and was coughing at night. His mom had to miss work, and Michael lost a day of school because he needed to be seen for a sick visit. It was determined that the medicine hadn't caused the rash, but a new bath soap had.

Stopping medicine abruptly interrupts treatment and puts children like Michael at risk to develop more problems, ranging from mild symptoms to a serious flare. Always call your health care professional and explain the problem so that another medicine can be tried or another cause of the side effect can be identified.

TAKING MEDICINE THE RIGHT TIME, THE RIGHT WAY

Medicines won't control asthma unless they are taken at the right time and in the right way.

Two-year-old Ryan needs two medicines, a daily controller medicine and a quick-relief kind for symptoms. He takes both medicines through a nebulizer, a machine that mixes medicine and air into a mist that's inhaled through a face mask or mouthpiece. But Ryan is a typically active toddler who doesn't like to sit still or wear a face mask. His frustrated parents feel badly when they have to hold him down to give him his daily nebulizer treatment, so they have given up the face mask and blow the mist of medicine in his face as best they can. They wonder if Ryan is getting any of the medicine. They have also become more concerned because his day care teacher reports that Ryan is wheezing during playtime.

When his parents take him in for a sick visit, they learn that virtually no medicine has been getting deep down into Ryan's lungs, which is why he is not doing well. The doctor and parents discuss strategies for getting him to wear the mask by making it a game, distracting him by reading a book, or giving him his treatment while he is asleep.

Older children present other challenges.

Thirteen-year-old Shakira has difficult-to-control asthma and is on numerous medicines. When her parents notice that she has symptoms, they ask her if she is taking her medicines. She assures them that she is. Meanwhile Shakira's doctor has been trying to figure out why she is not doing well. Shakira eventually admits that she often forgets to take her morning dose when she's rushing for school, but she hasn't told her parents because she worries they'll be angry with her.

When you take the time to have an honest conversation with teenagers, you find out that they have many reasons for not taking their medicines the way they should. Some of their reasons include: "I'm busy . . . I forget . . . I don't like the way the medicine makes me feel." But they often don't tell anyone because they're embarrassed about having asthma or about seeming different from other teens. Two other typical reasons: if they don't have symptoms, they don't understand the need for ongoing controller medicine; or they don't realize that it's important to take care of their lungs now so they'll be healthy years from now. (More about teenagers with asthma will be given in chapter 13.)

Children usually don't put asthma treatment at the top of their priority lists. They'd rather be out with their friends or playing a game. They'll remember their medicine when symptoms start to bother them, but it is difficult for them to remember to take it every day—*especially when they are feeling fine.*

Even when children are old enough to administer their own medicine, parents need to be aware of the correct techniques and timetables in order to supervise the way older children take their medicine. You don't want to feel as if you're a prison guard who must watch them each and every time. But let them know you believe the treatment is important by keeping a close eye to make sure that it is being taken correctly. You can support them in positive ways, such as praising them for remembering to take their medicine and trying not to sound accusatory when they forget.

RUNNING ON EMPTY

Even the most effective medicines can't control asthma if they run out. To keep your child's asthma under control, keep track of all medicines, know when they need to be refilled, and refill them before the container is empty.

> Sara is a four-year-old with asthma. About three weeks after starting an inhaled medicine called Flovent her asthma came under control. She stopped coughing at night, and she got over her last cold in less than a week. Two months later her symptoms returned with a vengeance, even though Sara's mother was giving her the medicine every day. It turned out that her mom used the same canister of Flovent for three months—long after the canister was empty. At Sara's follow-up appointment, Mom learned that the canister contains only enough medicine for one month.

When children skip medicine or use an empty inhaler, they run the risk of losing control of their asthma. These issues might seem like small details, but they are not uncommon. It is essential to be aware of them because they can make all the difference between controlling asthma or allowing it to spin out of control.

EDUCATION AND COMMUNICATION

The NIH guidelines set standards for health care professionals to educate patients about controlling asthma. Just as you expect your child's caregivers to provide prescriptions for medicine, you should also expect them to inform you (and your child if he's old enough to understand) about asthma. This information should come in two forms: general information about the disease and specific information tailored to your child. Although you can learn about asthma from organizations like the American Lung Association or Allergy & Asthma Network: Mothers of Asthmatics (see Resources), in books like this, and on the Internet, remember that only your child's physician or nurse practitioner can provide you with education that is individualized to meet your child's specific needs.

The national guidelines offer these key educational concepts, which your health care professional should review with you:

Basic facts about asthma: You should understand what the lungs do and what is wrong with the airways and lungs in someone with asthma. The airways are inflamed, irritated, and oversensitive on a chronic or ongoing basis. The airways overreact, and the muscles encircling them go into spasms that results in symptoms.

Roles of medicines: You should know the two categories of asthma medicines: (1) long-term controller medicines to prevent symptoms and attacks, and (2) quick-relief medicines to relieve symptoms and treat attacks.

In addition to this general information, it is essential to know the exact names (both brand names and generic names) of all your child's medicines, their strengths, what category they are (controller or quick-relief), how and when to take them, as well as how and when to refill them.

Skills: Whether your child is old enough to take her own medicines, you need to know how to administer each type correctly. Older children who are able to take their own medicine will need to practice and master the proper techniques, too.

Another important skill in keeping asthma under control is observation. When your child starts to cough and wheeze, you know that her asthma is acting up. You can monitor the state of her asthma by observing signs like her tolerance for activity, sleep patterns, and other symptoms. Some parents like to keep a written diary of these observations.

But these obvious signs don't always give the full picture because airway inflammation starts to increase before symptoms even appear. Sometimes the symptoms are mild—even though the airways are actually quite clogged from mucus and excess swelling. So observation isn't the only skill you'll need.

To help determine how open your child's lungs are, you may want to ask your doctor or nurse practitioner whether a *peak flow meter* is right for your child. A peak flow meter is a small, inexpensive device that measures how fast air moves out of your child's lungs when she exhales. It takes a little practice to learn how to use a peak flow meter properly—and what to do when it indicates a problem.

Triggers and environment: Parents need to understand the significance of identifying their child's asthma triggers and taking action to get rid of them or avoid them. To some parents, this may seem overwhelming at first because they assume they'll need to make major, expensive changes in their home. But that is rarely the case. Many simple ways to decrease and avoid triggers are suggested in chapter 10. Your child's asthma caregivers can help you prioritize which strategies can reduce exposure to triggers like dust, dander, smoke, and pollen.

Written asthma management plan: Every single child (and adult) with asthma should have a written treatment plan with specific instructions about how and when to take medicines, as well as how and when to increase medicine for symptoms and attacks. The plan should also spell out exactly what to do if the plan doesn't seem to help or if your child becomes worse. (More about a written plan will be given in chapter 7; see a sample written plan in Resources, pages 220–222.)

The written plan should guide you in recognizing signs that your child's asthma is getting out of control. Once your child starts to experience symptoms, try to identify the trigger and increase medicines as directed by your child's plan. The sooner you start extra treatments for symptoms and attacks, the more likely you are to get things under control quickly. The longer you wait to start, the more likely it is that your child's asthma could get out of control and result in a sick visit, emergency room treatment, or overnight stay in the hospital.

The written plan should cover all possibilities from what to do for common symptoms to an emergency situation. The plan should be written clearly and be readily available—on the refrigerator door or kitchen bulletin board. Tell baby-sitters and relatives where to find it when you aren't home, and be sure a responsible person at your child's school or day care center has a copy. A written plan not only provides vital information tailored to your child, but it also will help you feel that you have control in managing your child's asthma.

All of the education guidelines mentioned above are useful only if you and your child's doctor or nurse practitioner communicate about them. Ask questions at any time, not just when the plan is new or when your child has an unfamiliar symptom or side effect from medicine. Communicate with your child's health care professionals about all issues relating to her asthma. For example, if your insurance or prescription plan doesn't cover one of your child's medicines, let the doctor or nurse know so another medicine can be substituted or the insurance company contacted.

SATISFIED CUSTOMERS

Another important goal of therapy, according to the national guidelines, is one that is most often overlooked: you and your child should be satisfied with your asthma care. Has your child's doctor or nurse practitioner asked if you are satisfied with your child's care? If the question hasn't been asked, bring it up the next time you have an appointment. Open, two-way communication should include a discussion of the goals of asthma therapy and clear expectations of what control means for your child—not for all children in general, but for *your* individual child. For this to succeed, parents and professionals should be working as a team. You should feel comfortable asking questions, even ones that might seem "stupid." *There are no stupid questions* when it comes to your child's health.

When parents don't ask questions, many times a busy doctor or nurse will assume that parents understand what is going on and agree with the treatment plan. To ensure the best possible care for your child, you need to take responsibility by playing an active role.

COMMON SENSE

Remember: the best strategy for keeping asthma *under control* is to use common sense. Asthma cannot be cured, but control is a realistic, achievable goal. Parents need to use common sense in their relationship and communication with health care professionals. As a parent, you know your child best. You need to work with your child's physician or nurse practitioner to make sure that they learn whatever they need to know to match the treatment to your individual child and make it fit your family's lifestyle.

5

Asthma Medicines

A century ago, people with asthma smoked "asthma cigarettes" rolled from an herb called belladonna, or deadly nightshade. Modern medicine has come a long way since those early inhalers. Today a wide array of medicines is available to control and treat asthma effectively. But these therapies often are confusing because numerous generic and brand name medicines come in various doses and forms of delivery. Some are inhaled. Others come in pill or syrup form. To add to the confusion, your neighbor's child and your may child share virtually the same symptoms, yet different asthma medicines have been prescribed for each child. How is a parent to understand this pharmacopocia?

This chapter reviews current asthma medicines. Here is the essential starting point: asthma medicines fall into two basic categories.

1. *Controller* medicines
2. *Quick-relief* medicines

Doctors, nurses, and pharmaceutical companies use a variety of terms for these two groups. Controller medicine is also described as "preventive" or "maintenance" medicine. Quick-relief types are often called "rescue," "fast-relief," "fast-acting," or "as-needed" medicines. To be consistent and avoid confusion, the two categories are called *controller* and *quick-relief* medicines throughout this book.

Most asthma medicines can be taken by the inhaled route, although some can only be taken orally. Delivery devices—nebulizers, metered dose inhalers (MDIs), and dry powder inhalers (DPIs)—and the correct ways to use them will be discussed in greater detail in the next chapter. Allergy medicines and complementary therapies will be discussed at the end of this chapter.

CONTROLLER MEDICINES

Most parents don't hesitate to give medicine when children have symptoms. But it may be more difficult to justify medicine when symptoms are absent. "He's doing fine—he's running around, not coughing, not wheezing. Why does he need it?" some parents wonder. This dilemma is more pronounced when a child has a chronic illness like asthma that requires daily medicines—even when symptoms aren't present. Chronic conditions often present a "Three Bears" challenge: what's "not enough," "too much," or "just right"?

Parents, physicians, and nurse practitioners are all working toward the same goal—to administer the least amount of medicine required to control a child's asthma. Health care professionals write prescriptions, but they recognize that parents play the most important role. As a parent, you are the day-to-day supervisor when it comes to dosing the medicines. For that reason, it is critical for parents to understand the keys to good asthma control—a clear understanding how medicines work, their possible side effects, and the risk of *not* treating between asthma episodes. If you have this knowledge and work as a team with your child's health care providers, you will be able to make informed decisions about your child's treatment.

As the name implies, controller medicines are used to control asthma by preventing symptoms. They are given on a regular basis, often twice daily, even when a child is symptom-free. They are *not* meant to relieve symptoms when they arise.

Because asthma's underlying problem is airway inflammation, a treatment plan for a child whose asthma is mild persistent or worse (see chapter 2) should include an anti-inflammatory medicine. Some controller medicines are not considered anti-inflammatory, but they do help control asthma when combined with anti-inflammatory medicines.

Controller medicines must be used daily if you want to keep your child symptom-free. You may not see the benefit of a controller medicine right away, but over several weeks your child will have fewer, less intense symptoms as the medicine gradually reduces airway inflammation.

Children with persistent asthma—those with frequent symptoms—should be on controller medicines. Some children who don't have persistent asthma but have difficulty controlling flares or have symptoms brought on by exercise or physical activity may also benefit by controller medicines. (More about exercise-induced asthma will be given in chapter 11.) For these children, controller medicines may be prescribed or changed seasonally, such as during the spring and fall allergy seasons or the winter viral season.

Most controller medicines must be taken for two to six weeks to produce any noticeable benefit. Giving medicine every day is not easy, especially when you do not see immediate improvement in your child. But try to be patient and stick with it because it will pay off in fewer, less intense symptoms over the long run.

Types of controller medicines are described below.

Inhaled Corticosteroids (ICSs)

These medicines are the most effective controller medicines available to date. The National Institutes of Health considers inhaled corticosteroids (ICSs) to be the preferred first-line therapy in children and adults with persistent asthma. They are the gold standard against which other controller medicines are compared.

Inhaled corticosteroids have several important benefits. They prevent medical visits, school absences, limited activity, use of quick-relief medicines and oral corticosteroids, hospitalization, and even death.

Parents are often concerned about side effects related to ICS use. ICSs are often confused with anabolic steroids, which are used to build up muscles. ICSs are *not* the same, and side effects are much less worrisome.

Inhaled corticosteroids take time to work. Depending on the individual preparation, they may take several days or several weeks to have full effect. They are not meant to be used for quick relief of symptoms or just before exercise or exposure to allergens. Regular use of ICSs, however, will make asthma triggers less likely to cause symptoms by decreasing the underlying inflammation that occurs in even the mildest forms of asthma. In other words, a child's lungs will be in better shape to resist triggers if ICSs are used regularly.

Preparations available as ICS include the following medicines, listed in both brand and generic names:

Advair (fluticasone plus salmeterol)

Aerobid (flunisolide)

Azmacort (triamcinolone)

Beclovent (beclomethasone)

Flovent (fluticasone)

Pulmicort Respules (budesonide inhalation suspension)

Pulmicort Turbuhaler (budesonide)

Vanceril (beclomethasone)

QVAR (beclomethasone)

Fluticasone (Flovent) and budesonide (Pulmicort) are called "second-generation" inhaled corticosteroids because they are the newest ICSs available. They are considered safer yet more effective than some of the older preparations. QVAR is the same medicine as the older Beclovent and Vanceril, but it is used with a new nonaerosol propellant that will not harm the ozone layer. Since the force of the spray and size of the inhaled particles are different from earlier formulations, more medicine gets deposited throughout the lungs and less is swallowed.

Pulmicort Turbuhaler and Advair are dry powder medicines inhaled directly into the lungs through the mouth. Devices used for administration crush the tablet form of the medicine into very fine particles that can be inhaled. Since they are not aerosols, they do not harm the ozone layer.

Side Effects of Inhaled Corticosteroids

Moderate to high doses of inhaled corticosteroids may cause a child's growth rate to slow down slightly, but it's usually less than one-half inch during the first year of use. By the second year, the growth rate will be back to normal. Even when this does occur, children catch up and reach their normal predicted adult height. Weight and sexual development are not affected.

Other possible side effects of inhaled corticosteroids are hoarseness and thrush (a yeast infection of mouth). By using a spacer device (see below) and rinsing the mouth after each use, you can decrease these effects.

The best way to minimize side effects of a corticosteroid is to deliver it directly to the airways, where it is most effective. Proper delivery to the airways reduces the amount of medicine that enters the bloodstream, which could cause side effects. Because much of an inhaled medicine goes down the throat and is swallowed, there is always a chance that some medicine will enter the bloodstream.

When some of the medicine is swallowed, it gets into the intestinal tract, is processed by the liver, and sent into the bloodstream. When the swallowed medicine is active, it is described medically as having "a high oral bioavailability." Some older inhaled corticosteroids (like beclomethasone) had high oral bioavailability and were therefore more prone to causing side effects. Newer inhaled corticosteroids, such as Flovent and Pulmicort, are not very active when swallowed because the liver turns them into inactive medicine.

Spacer devices help to reduce oral intake. A spacer (such as Aerochamber, Optichamber, and Inspirease) decreases the amount of medicine that is swallowed when using a metered dose inhaler (MDI). A metered dose inhaler releases an exact, measured amount of medicine from an aerosol canister each time the child takes a puff. As a result, side effects associated with oral intake of the inhaled medicines are decreased.

Much smaller amounts of inhaled medicine can enter the bloodstream through the blood vessels in the lungs. But if the dose is high enough, even the newer inhaled corticosteroids may enter the bloodstream this way. It is important to remember that children who need such high doses have more severe asthma and that the side effects are still far fewer than with an oral steroid. Keeping the dose at the lowest amount that adequately controls the asthma will minimize any side effects.

Long-Acting Bronchodilators

These medicines open the airways, but they do not act quickly enough to be used as quick-relief medicine when symptoms arise. They don't wear off as fast as quick-relief medicine and can provide benefit for about twelve hours. Since they are not anti-inflammatory, they should never be used *alone.*

Long-acting bronchodilators are available in the following preparations:

Foradil Aerolizer (formoterol)

Serevent (salmeterol) inhaler or Diskus

Advair Diskus (Serevent plus Flovent)

Foradil, Serevent Diskus, and Advair are all dry powder inhalers. Serevent also comes in a metered dose inhaler.

These long-acting bronchodilators can help prevent exercise-induced symptoms, particularly for children who exercise for more than a few hours at a time. To prevent an exercise-induced bronchospasm (EIB), salmeterol should be given thirty to sixty minutes before starting to exercise.

"Steroid Sparing"

Combined with inhaled corticosteroids, long-acting bronchodilators are very effective in controlling asthma symptoms and improving lung function. In fact, your child may need about half the dose of inhaled corticosteroid if your physician combines the inhaled corticosteroids with a long-acting bronchodilator. In other words, the dose of corticosteroid can be half of what would otherwise be required to control asthma. This is called "steroid sparing." Since inhaled corticosteroids at higher doses may have side effects, "sparing" is a way to minimize the steroid dose.

Long-acting bronchodilators are unlikely to cause side effects, such as increased heart rate and muscle tremors seen with the short-acting bronchodilators, which will be discussed later in this chapter.

"Sparing" can be done in single or combined ways, depending on which medicine your child takes. Advair combines the corticosteroid and long-acting bronchodilator in one dose. Foradil has to be taken in addition to the inhaled corticosteroid. If a child cannot use the Advair Diskus properly, he could use the Flovent and Serevent inhalers separately.

Mast Cell Stabilizers

Mast cells are a type of inflammatory cell in the airways. Mast cell stabilizers are a class of nonsteroid controller medicines that reduce the release of inflammation-causing chemicals from these cells. Their safety has been well established. In fact, even pregnant women and young infants can use them safely. Mast cell stabilizers include cromolyn (Intal), available in an inhaled or nebulized form, and nedocromil (Tilade), available only in an inhaled form.

Mast cell stabilizers can also be given twenty to thirty minutes before exposure to prevent allergen and exercise-induced symptoms. In general, with the improved safety of newer, low-dose inhaled corticosteroids, the development of a nebulized corticosteroid (Pulmicort), and the availability of a more effective, less cumbersome nonsteroid class of controller medicine (anti-leukotrienes), the role of mast cell stabilizers has been significantly reduced.

Theophylline

Theophylline is an older bronchodilator that was used frequently for both controller and quick-relief use with symptom flares. It is available in syrups, pills, and injectable forms. It does not have significant anti-inflammatory effects, so it became less popular as a preventive treatment when the role of inflammation was recognized. Theophylline is related to caffeine. Side effects (abdominal pain, nausea, vomiting, headaches, tremors, and increased heart rate) are common. High doses can cause serious side effects, so blood levels need to be monitored. With the high incidence of side effects and availability of safer alternatives, this medicine is used infrequently today.

Anti-leukotrienes

During allergic reactions, a naturally occurring chemical called histamine is released in the nose, eyes, and skin (see chapter 3). Another group of chemicals called *leukotrienes* is also released during allergic reactions. These chemicals are considered to be very important contributors to asthma symptoms.

A class of medicine called anti-leukotrienes blocks leukotrienes and can improve asthma control. Anti-leukotrienes can be used as an addition or alternative to inhaled corticosteroids. They are very safe, with side effects reported as similar to a placebo or sugar pill. Anti-leukotrienes are not as effective as inhaled corticosteroids. But like long-acting bronchodilators, they may allow the inhaled corticosteroids dose to be reduced, but to a lesser degree than with long-acting bronchodilators.

Anti-leukotrienes aren't usually effective as a controller medicine when used alone, except in milder forms of asthma. Anti-leukotrienes can have the advantage of helping to minimize other common allergy symptoms, especially when they are combined with antihistamines. They may also be helpful in preventing exercise- or allergen-induced bronchospasms.

Anti-leukotriene preparations are available as

Singulair (montelukast)

Accolate (zafirlukast)

Accolate is available only as a tablet and should be taken on an empty stomach twice a day. Singulair is available as regular or chewable tablets and should be taken daily at bedtime.

QUICK-RELIEF MEDICINE

Even when your child is routinely using a controller medicine, unexpected triggers can appear and set off symptoms, so your child should always have a quick-relief medicine available to use as soon as symptoms arise. If quick-relief medicine is used in this way—but not overused—it can prevent symptoms from developing into a full-blown flare.

As the term implies, quick-relief medicine is given to relieve asthma symptoms and is used on an as-needed basis but *only* when needed. Ideally, quick-relief medicine is used less than once a week on an average.

Quick-relief medicines are most commonly categorized as bronchodilators because they work by rapidly opening up—dilating—tight, constricted airways in a mechanism called bronchodilation. The short-acting bronchodilators are the principal class of medicines that are considered quick-relief medicines. Bronchodilators used today are selective—that is, the effect of the medicine is targeted for certain receptors in the lungs. In the 1960s, these medicines became available in metered dose inhaler (MDI) format. They are the most widely prescribed medicines for the treatment of asthma in both children and adults. More than 70 percent of all prescriptions written by pediatricians for asthma medicines are for quick-relief bronchodilator medicines.

Yet excessive use and overreliance on short-acting bronchodilators is often a warning sign that a child's asthma is flaring out of control. If your child requires frequent use of bronchodilators, this is a signal that a more effective regimen for controller medicines is required.

Although there is no controversy about using bronchodilators off and on to relieve asthma symptoms or prevent exercise-induced symptoms, there are major concerns about their use on a regular basis two or more times per day for treatment of chronic asthma. Quick-relief bronchodilators are most important as a first step in any asthma management plan, but parents must be very careful about how often their child uses these medicines.

Most canisters of quick-relief bronchodilators contain 200 puffs of medicine, and a canister should last several months. If a canister lasts less than three months, this should be a warning sign that the underlying asthma is not well controlled. Any child who uses more than two canisters of a bronchodilator over the course of a year should also be on some type of controller medicine, at least for part of the year when the symptoms are most significant. The frequency of bronchodilator use serves as a very useful indicator of the severity of the asthma and of the need for additional controller (anti-inflammatory) medicines.

Albuterol (the generic name) or other related medicines are the most frequently prescribed quick-relief medicines. Different brands are sold under various names, such as Proventil, Ventolin, and Maxair. These medicines work very quickly—usually within five minutes—when given in the inhaled form. Albuterol can also be administered in an oral preparation as syrup or pill. The inhaled form can be administered with a metered dose inhaler, used with a spacer to ensure proper delivery of the medicine, or via a nebulizer, a machine that mixes medicine with air to form a mist that is inhaled. The nebulizer is usually best for infants and young children. It involves using a mouthpiece or mask to deliver the medicine directly into the airways. (See chapter 6 for the correct way to use these delivery devices.)

When children are hospitalized for asthma treatment, albuterol is almost always given with a nebulizer to deliver the medicine effectively. It is also common practice in many settings to deliver the medicine by nebulizer when youngsters have a flare triggered by a viral infection. When the medicine is administered in an inhaled form, it goes directly to the lungs and isn't absorbed through the gastrointestinal tract and, therefore, leads to fewer side effects.

Side Effects of Quick-Relief Medicine

The most common side effects include jitteriness, headaches, and muscle tremors. Or the heart may be stimulated with excessive use and palpitations. These side effects can often be limited by lowering the dose of the bronchodilator as well as decreasing the frequency of use.

A new form of albuterol may have fewer side effects but it is too early to tell for sure. It is called *levalbuterol* (sold under the name of Xopenex). Levalbuterol is currently available only in a preparation that can be used in a nebulizer. It is not yet available in an inhaler form or in an oral preparation. The levalbuterol form is presently available in three different dosages. The decision on the appropriate dosage for a child depends on the age of the child as well as the severity of the asthma.

Anticholinergics

A small percentage of children may not tolerate the use of quick-relief bronchodilators. For that group, another medicine called Atrovent is often used. (Its generic name is ipratropium bromide.) This medicine falls into a category known as an "anticholinergic." As the quick-relief brochodilators relax the airway's smooth muscle, anticholinergics work to relax muscle tone. Some health care practitioners simultaneously administer albuterol and Atrovent together for an acute flare of asthma when a child is hospitalized. This combination treatment plan is common enough that the medicines can be obtained in their combined form (Duonebs when administered in a nebulizer form and Combivent when administered in an inhaled form). Since the medicines work via different pathways in the lungs, they have an added effect on relieving airway obstruction, which is why they can be administered together. Atrovent is used much more frequently in adults with chronic obstructive pulmonary disease than it is in children with asthma.

"BURST THERAPY"

If a child is having a significant flare and is not responding well to the use of the quick-relief medicines, intravenous or oral corticosteroids will often be used to treat moderate to severe flares. They will prevent the flare from becoming worse, help speed recovery, and prevent relapse. They do not open lungs but rather clear out the significant mucus that results from the inflammation associated with a severe, prolonged asthma attack. When steroids are administered in this fashion it is often referred to as *burst therapy* because the medicine is often given for three to ten days and then discontinued. Burst therapy is a short-term treatment for a significant flare of the asthma and should not be confused with the use of inhaled steroids as a controller therapy.

Intravenous or oral corticosteroids used in burst therapy are a much higher dose than is administered through an inhaler. They should not be used on a daily basis as part of a basic asthma management plan because long-term use of oral steroids can be associated with significant side effects over time. This does not occur with the inhaled steroids, however.

Some physicians believe that the newer preparations of the inhaled steroids (fluticasone and budesonide) are more potent and selective than the first generation of the inhaled steroids. Significant flares can also be treated effectively with "high" dose inhaled steroids for one week instead of administering oral steroids. Many children respond better to a doubling or tripling of their dose of inhaled steroids when they begin to experience a flare than resorting to oral steroids. The moodiness and increased appetite that are often associated with oral steroids is very rarely seen with inhaled steroids, even when the dosage is doubled or tripled from the usual dosage.

An effective treatment for a flare often includes the aggressive short-term use of quick-relief medicines, as well as an increased dose of inhaled steroids for one week or oral steroids for a few days if a child continues to show signs of persistent, significant symptoms. Once the flare is well controlled, the quick-relief medicine will be decreased accordingly.

One common misconception is that children will become dependent on the use of these medicines if used frequently. Excessive use of the quick-relief medicine is a warning sign that the underlying process of asthma is not well controlled and is not a result of the use of the medicines.

Oral Corticosteroids

Oral corticosteroids take about six hours to have full effect. But once they begin to work, they help control the asthma flare. They get rid of the inflammation that has built up during a flare. They also make the lungs more responsive to the short-acting bronchodilator, so it is important to continue the bronchodilator while on the oral corticosteroid until symptoms subside. Oral corticosteroids are generally prescribed for three to ten days with each flare. Some children will require a longer course. Others need to stay on a low dose every day or every other day as a controller medicine for severe asthma. Taking the lowest possible dose every other morning can minimize side effects.

Many preparations of oral corticosteroids are available in pill and syrup forms. The strength of each varies, so be sure to follow the directions on each new prescription. Do not assume the dose will be the same number of pills or teaspoons as prescribed for your child in the past. Unfortunately, this medicine tastes bitter, so many children resist it. If they cannot swallow pills very well, the tablet may taste bitter on their tongues.

These medicines are available in these forms and brands:

Tablets	**Syrups (prednisolone)**
prednisone (Deltasone)	Orapred
methylprednisolone (Medrol)	Pediapred
	Prelone

Sometimes an oral corticosteroid is prescribed with instructions to lower the dose gradually each day when prescribed for longer time periods. One reason for tapering off the dose is based on the fact that the body makes its own corticosteroids to handle stress. Tapering the medicine is only necessary if the treatment course is two weeks or longer in order to allow the body a chance to produce its own steroids. Inhaled corticosteroids may be used to prevent recurrence of symptoms once the oral corticosteroids are stopped.

Oral corticosteroids can sometimes produce side effects. When they occur, it is usually from high doses or prolonged use. Possible side effects include fluid retention (puffiness), thinning of the bones, irritation or bleeding of the stomach, high blood pressure, glaucoma, and cataracts. Oral corticosteroids may also impair the body's ability to fight some infections. A single brief course doesn't usually cause these serious side effects; however, increased appetite, weight gain, mood change, and upset stomach may occur.

Some long-term effects may appear with multiple, brief courses of oral corticosteroids, but exactly how many brief courses are safe is not completely known. The much safer inhaled steroids, used as controller medicines, can greatly reduce the chance of needing oral corticosteroids.

ALLERGY MEDICINES

Many children with asthma also need allergy medicine. Treating allergy symptoms in the nose has been shown to help control asthma and prevent flares. One often-overlooked function of the nose is to warm, moisturize, and filter the air we breathe. Some children with allergies cannot breathe through their noses so they inhale colder, drier, dirtier air through their mouths, which can aggravate their asthma. Antihistamines with or without decongestants and nasal steroids may be prescribed to control allergies. If allergies are not adequately controlled, allergy shots may be given to make your child's body less allergic.

COMPLEMENTARY THERAPIES FOR ASTHMA

About one of every three Americans has tried herbal medicines, acupuncture, traditional Chinese medicine, homeopathy, yoga, chiropractic manipulation, high-dose vitamins and minerals, and relaxation techniques. These types of complementary medicine, also called "alternative" or "integrative" medicine, have not been studied and evaluated with controlled studies as rigorously as traditional Western medicines. But alternative approaches are coming into mainstream medicine. At least seventy-five medical schools—including University of Pennsylvania, Harvard, Yale, Johns Hopkins, and Columbia—now offer courses in complementary medicine.

Because complementary therapies have become so widely used in recent years, parents may wonder if they could help relieve their child's asthma symptoms. The following review of the most common alternative therapies is based on published studies of their merit.

Chiropractic manipulation was not found to be helpful for asthma in any study. The results were more mixed for **acupuncture.** Five studies found that acupuncture was not beneficial, and eight studies found that it worked better than nothing. But in all studies, acupuncture didn't work as well as albuterol in treating asthma symptoms.

Yoga was studied in conjunction with standard asthma medicines, such as inhaled corticosteroids. Individuals who did yoga or relaxation therapies noted an improvement in their asthma symptoms (fewer, milder symptoms and improved lung function). Yoga did not replace standard therapies but was added to them in these studies.

Many modern medicines are derived from herbal therapies. The advantage of modern medicine over herbs, however, is that potential benefits are maximized, while potential serious side effects are minimized. One of the most common **herbal therapies** is *Ma huang*, whose active ingredient is distantly related to albuterol, the common quick-relief medicine for asthma. Its active ingredient, L-ephedrine, is also very similar to Sudafed, an over-the-counter decongestant. High doses of ephedrine are known to have adverse effects that include high blood pressure, rapid heart rate, nervousness, headache, insomnia, dizziness, seizure, stroke, and fatal myocardial infarction (heart attack).

The second most common herb used to treat asthma is *Atropa belladonna* (deadly nightshade). Its active ingredient is atropine, which is similar to the active ingredient in Atrovent, a common medicine for other lung diseases. Belladonna was once burned in cigarettes, referred to as "asthma cigarettes." These primitive "inhalers" were a popular treatment for asthma and other respiratory conditions in Europe and North America in the early part of the twentieth century. Potential side effects include dry mouth, dangerously low heart rate, nausea, and headache.

Ginkgo biloba is used around the world for a variety of illnesses. The main ingredients, ginkgolides, may prevent twitchy airways or coughing. Side effects of ginkgo include nausea, vomiting, diarrhea, salivation, anorexia, headache, dizziness, ringing in the ears, and allergic reactions. No controlled studies have shown a benefit of ginkgo biloba for asthma.

Licorice root is used to prevent cough and increase the clearance of mucus. Its active ingredients include glycyrrhizin, which may prolong the action of steroids. No controlled studies of licorice have been conducted for asthma in humans, so it's important to discuss with your child's physician any complementary medicines you are using, particularly in the case of an herb like licorice, which has an effect of increasing steroid potency.

Saiboku-tois is the most popular anti-asthmatic herbal treatment used in Japanese Kampo medicines. In China, it is called *chaipu-tang*. It is supposed to decrease the metabolism of steroids, and it therefore increases the potency and effectiveness of inhaled steroids. It also increases the risk of side effects from inhaled steroids, but when taken by itself, it has not been found to be as effective as inhaled steroids.

Tylophora indica is an herb used commonly in the Ayurvedic system of medicine practiced in India. It is claimed to increase mucus clearing and is also recognized as a bronchodilator similar to a quick-relief medicine like albuterol. The effectiveness of this medicine is quite variable, with helpful effects in one study and no effects in other studies.

Several studies have examined high-dose *vitamin C* in the treatment of asthma. Similar to many herbal therapies, vitamin C's effects vary, with some studies reporting beneficial effects and other studies reporting none.

Interestingly, many current Western medicines are based on previous complementary medicines. An old therapy for asthma, for example, was ground adrenal glands of animals. Adrenal glands have steroids and albuterol-like compounds that have similarities to the inhaled steroids and bronchodilators used today.

Many herbal supplements can be safe when used appropriately, but known and potential risks of such compounds do exist. A misconception exists that herbs are safe because they come from plants. The chemical makeup of plants and herbs is sophisticated, and many are toxic. Often other medicines, such as steroids and aspirinlike medicines, are added to these herbal supplements to improve their effect and potential side-effects. Other factors can cause problems, including inconsistent dosing and drug interactions.

There is also no licensing body for the practice of herbal medicine in the United States. Most herbs are marketed as dietary supplements and are not regulated by the FDA. There is no guarantee, therefore, of quality or consistency. The advantage of traditional Western medicines is that they are controlled, regulated, and given in more palatable formats.

It is also important to remember that alternative medicines can interact with standard medicines for asthma, so it is important to talk to your child's physician or nurse practitioner about any herbal medicines that your child may be taking.

FUTURE DIRECTIONS FOR THE PREVENTION AND TREATMENT OF ASTHMA

Many treatments continue to be developed to fight airway inflammation found in asthma. New approaches are aimed at cells, chemicals, and antibodies responsible for allergic inflammation. Some of these involve genetically engineering antibodies to affect parts of the immune system. Some may involve injections and may be rather expensive. As a result, they may initially be indicated for individuals on high doses of corticosteroids or those with symptoms despite traditional therapies. Other treatments are being developed to prevent or alter the natural history of asthma by introducing immune-modifying treatments in early childhood.

Despite the possible side effects of some of these medicines—standard, traditional, and complementary—the biggest asthma risk is the disease itself. In some children, untreated inflammation can lead to irreversible changes in the airways. Asthma is the most common cause of hospitalization in children, and each year about 200 American children die from asthma. Even children with mild asthma are at risk for any or all these complications. Fortunately, taking medicine appropriately can minimize all the risks.

6

Medicine the Right Way

A sthma medicines come in several different forms. When you think of medicine, you probably think of liquids or pills, but only a few asthma medicines are taken by mouth. Asthma is best treated by *inhaled* medicine because it goes directly where it needs to work—the lungs—rather than into the intestinal tract, the bloodstream, and throughout the whole body.

This chapter focuses on the correct ways to use inhaled medicines and the proper methods of taking care of them. One of the most important issues in controlling asthma is matching the treatment to the individual child. That means not only giving the most appropriate medicine, but also being sure its delivery device is used the right way for it to work effectively.

Treatment for asthma comes primarily in three types of inhaled medicines: *metered dose inhalers* (MDIs), *dry powder inhalers* (DPIs), and *nebulizers*.

METERED DOSE INHALERS (MDIs) AND SPACERS

MDIs have been used for asthma and other lung diseases for several decades. These small, plastic, handheld devices contain medicine in an aerosol canister. When sprayed, the inhaler expels an exact, measured dose of medicine—either a controller or a quick-relief type.

The MDI container also contains a chemical propellant that delivers the medicine very fast. If you've ever put an MDI in your mouth and sprayed it, you have felt a wet, cold spray in your mouth and throat. But the problem with feeling that spray is that the medicine landed in your mouth and throat instead of going deep down your windpipe and into the lungs where it needs to work.

In the past, many children used an MDI by itself, but today it is highly recommended that a *spacer* be added to the MDI for a more effective treatment. A spacer—also called a "holding chamber"—holds and slows down the spray so a child can inhale a slower, deeper breath. When a child uses a spacer with a one-way valve, he can't exhale air into the spacer, so he's able to inhale all the medicine deep into his lungs. (Other kinds, without a one-way valve are available, but the one-way valve type is preferable.) He will not feel a wet cold spray in his mouth. When using a spacer with an MDI, a child should be reminded to take a slow, deep breath and hold it for ten seconds.

A number of different brands of spacers are on the market. They require a prescription, and prices vary. Most brands have a mouthpiece that adults, teenagers, and children as young as five or six years old can use correctly and consistently. Spacers are also made with a face mask for babies and toddlers.

Many children, particularly those with mild asthma, have been using MDIs without spacers for some time. They and their parents may assume that the MDI alone is enough, but it can present problems, as this fifteen-year-old discovered:

> David had been taking Flovent 44 as his controller medicine without
> a spacer for over two years. He used it when he was supposed to,

every morning and every night, but he still had symptoms during colds and exercise. When his nurse practitioner asked David how he knows when the inhaler is empty and how often he refills it, David said that he asks his mother for a refill whenever the inhaler feels empty and no spray comes out. The nurse explained that David's particular MDI comes with 120 "actuations" (individual doses of medicine). That means that if David takes four puffs a day (two puffs twice a day) for thirty days, one Flovent MDI should last a month.

The nurse practitioner also urged David to get a new MDI every month even if he still feels liquid in the canister and sees spray come out. After 120 puffs of medicine have been taken, there may still be some liquid (preservative and propellant) in the canister. It may not "feel empty," but it contains no medicine.

Not all medicines that come as MDIs contain 120 doses per canister or are prescribed for four puffs a day. Be sure you understand how often your child is supposed to use the MDI/spacer and check the individual canister for its number of total doses.

Sometimes parents worry that older children, who are allowed to monitor their own medicine, are taking it too often or too little. A rule of thumb to remember is that quick-relief medicine, such as albuterol dispensed as an MDI, should contain 200 doses. If a child's asthma is well controlled, a refill will be needed every six months. If your child is using more than this, or is taking albuterol twice a week or more, discuss this with your child's health care professional.

After David's nurse practitioner explained this, he and his mother decided to keep better track by writing down the date on the kitchen calendar each time he starts a new MDI—both controller and quick-relief medicines. This not only reminds them to call the pharmacy for a refill before the medicine runs out, but it also helps them both be aware of how much quick-relief medicine David is using so they can keep an eye on over-use or under-use.

Instead of increasing his dose of Flovent to 110, David's nurse practitioner considered two options. One was to continue the Flovent 44, but teach David how to use a spacer and explain that it will also help him get better relief by controlling airway inflammation and preventing symptoms. The second option was to switch him to a dry powder inhaler

(DPI), which does not require a spacer but does require learning a different administration technique.

DRY POWDER INHALERS (DPIS)

DPIs are the newest device on the market. They deliver medicine to the airways as a dry powder. Taking medicine with a DPI is quick—it takes less than a minute to take a dose. DPIs require no special care except to keep them dry. Most children older than five years of age are able to learn the administration technique. But regardless of a child's age, parents still must pay attention to make sure their child performs the correct technique consistently.

If your child has previously used an MDI/spacer and is just beginning to use a DPI, be sure she understands that the DPI is used differently—she must be able to take in *a fast, deep breath* rather than the slow, deep breath required by an MDI/spacer. With both an MDI and DPI, a child should hold the breath for ten seconds after inhaling the puff of medicine.

Since not all asthma medicines are available in the DPI form, your child needs to know the proper technique for more than one device—in other words, she'll have to become a switch-hitter and learn when and how to use at least two or maybe even three techniques for taking different inhaled medicines.

You may wonder what difference it makes whether she inhales a fast, deep breath or a slow, deep one. The answer lies simply in the fact that an MDI contains a chemical propellant that expels the spray very fast. As discussed earlier, the spacer holds the puff of medicine so, as a child slowly inhales it, the medicine is more effectively delivered deep down into her lungs. DPIs, however, do not contain a propellant. A DPI can only work and get deep down to her lower airways if she takes a fast, deep breath.

There are currently three DPI devices on the market in the United States:

The *Diskus* is available with either salmeterol (Serevent) or fluticasone in combination with salmeterol (Advair). Both medicines are long-term controller medicines. If a child uses Advair, for example, she would also have to be able to take quick-relief medicine by MDI with a spacer or nebulizer (discussed later in this chapter). The Diskus comes with a dose counter.

Another controller medicine, *budesonide*, is an inhaled corticosteroid that comes in two forms: Turbuhaler is a dry powder, and Respules are a liquid solution for a nebulizer. If a child is on the Pulmicort Turbuhaler, she'll need to take her quick-relief medicine (albuterol) by MDI/spacer or nebulizer. The Turbuhaler has an indicator to let you know when it's running empty.

A third DPI device is the *Aerolizer* that contains formoterol (Foradil), which is similar to salmeterol. Both formoterol and salmeterol are long-term controller medicines, but they are not anti-inflammatory medicines. If formoterol or salmeterol is prescribed for your child, she will also need both an anti-inflammatory medicine and a quick-relief medicine. The Aerolizer is loaded with a one-dose capsule for each use so it's easy to check that the whole dose has been taken. When you discard the capsule after taking the dose, you can see whether or not the capsule is empty.

It's important to understand that there may be variations in how different DPIs are used. For example, the Pulmicort device is twisted one way, then the other. With Advair, the device is opened and then a lever is pulled. For both of these, a child must breathe in quickly and deeply once the tablet is crushed, and the medicine is deposited into his lungs.

Advair has a slightly sweet taste, and Pulmicort does not. Often parents of children taking Pulmicort worry that their children aren't getting the medicine because they cannot taste anything. Your physician or nurse practitioner can assess whether your child is capable of inhaling deeply enough to draw the powder into her lungs. These devices are very easy to use, and they have counters that tell how many doses are left.

NEBULIZERS

A nebulizer is a machine that uses an air compressor to mix liquid medicine with air and form a mist that is inhaled through a mouthpiece or face mask. (Technically, the "machine" part is the air compressor, and the "nebulizer" is the tubing with medicine cup. "Nebulizer" is used here in its broader, more common meaning as the whole device.)

When children are first diagnosed with asthma, many times they are treated using a nebulizer. After this initial experience, parents may think that a nebulizer is the most preferred way to administer medicine. Nebulizers are just one way to give asthma medicines. Other devices may be more effective and less cumbersome.

While many parents and even some health care professionals think that the nebulizer is the best way to give asthma medicine, research has not shown that to be true. Many children, especially infants and toddlers, don't seem to improve on a nebulizer because their caretakers have not been taught the proper technique for giving a nebulizer treatment. Proper technique is just as important when medicine is given by nebulizer as it is when given by an MDI/spacer or a DPI.

Sometimes parents observe incorrect techniques for nebulizer treatments administered by the "blow-by method," which is holding the tube, with mist coming out of it, in the child's face. This technique is often used when a child won't cooperate by wearing a mask or is too young to use a mouthpiece. The main problem with the blow-by method is that very little medicine gets down deep into the lungs where it is needed, and most of the medicine is wasted.

When a mouthpiece or face mask is used with a nebulizer, it's important to be sure that your child takes slow, deep breaths and holds each breath for five to ten seconds before inhaling the next breath. If a child is allowed to breathe normally during the nebulizer treatment, the medicine won't get into the airways effectively. Another problem with using a nebulizer for an infant or toddler is that, while you may get him to wear the face mask, he is also crying and taking fast, shallow breaths rather than the proper deep, slower breaths. (See chapter 12 for more about infants and toddlers.)

Even when the proper technique is used, nebulizer treatments take about ten minutes or longer. Another drawback is that a nebulizer is not easily portable. This is an important issue because families are constantly on the go, and children may need to take medicine at day care or school. A nebulizer is cumbersome to carry along with everything else that children need.

Instructions for nebulizer equipment may differ from model to model, so if your child uses a nebulizer, be sure that you keep and follow the manufacturer's instructions that come with the machine. Proper administration technique is absolutely essential if you want the nebulizer medicine to work. Here's an example of what can happen if the technique is incorrect:

> When three-year-old Ramon went for a checkup, he was not doing well. As his long-term control treatment, he was on Pulmicort Respules 0.25 mg. Ramon's mother reported that he'd been having lots of symptoms during the day when he played and at night.
>
> His pediatrician considered increasing Ramon's dose to 0.5 mg, but before writing the prescription she asked his mother about how she was giving him the medicine. It turned out that Ramon wouldn't wear the face mask so his parents had been blowing the medicine in his face. The doctor explained that this was undoubtedly why Ramon wasn't inhaling enough medicine. She suggested distracting Ramon during the treatment by reading him a story or giving the treatment with a face mask when he is asleep. By the next visit, Ramon's symptoms had diminished without increasing his dose of medicine.

Nebulizers should not be shared. If you have more than one child who uses a nebulizer, be sure that each child has her own air compressor and nebulizer tubing with medicine cup. Nebulizer equipment is sometimes covered by insurance; ask your provider. If you have questions about whether your child's nebulizer is working properly, call the durable medical equipment company that provided the machine. The company's name and phone number should be on the machine or in the operating instructions. While nebulizers have drawbacks, they do work well for those children who are willing to put on the mask or put the mouthpiece in their mouths to take their treatments. Many youngsters will read, play a quiet game, or sleep through a nebulizer treatment.

TAKING MEDICINE AND EQUIPMENT WITH YOU

Whenever your child has health care appointments, take along her medicine and equipment so that any questions about the condition of her devices can be looked into during the visit. This should not be difficult to remember because you should have your child's quick-relief medicine and spacer with you wherever you go in case symptoms appear. By taking your child's treatment devices to regular medical appointments, you can also ask your health care professional to make sure your child is using them correctly. If your child has been using them incorrectly, the proper method can be demonstrated.

Whenever you have questions about your child's medicine use, effectiveness, or technique, don't hesitate to ask your physician or nurse practitioner. As you know by now, medicine and its delivery methods can be confusing. Some medicines come in more than one formulation, while others don't. Albuterol, for example, comes in liquid form that can be given by nebulizer or an MDI with a spacer. The MDI/spacer is smaller, lighter, and easier than a nebulizer to take along wherever your child goes. And an MDI/spacer is a quick way to take medicine. A child can take two medicines—an inhaled corticosteroid and albuterol—one after the other in less time than it takes for one nebulizer treatment, and that's not counting the time it takes to set up the nebulizer first and clean it afterward.

WHAT YOU NEED TO KNOW

The bottom line when it comes to giving asthma medicines the right way is your role and responsibility as parent. Here's a checklist of what every parent of a child with asthma should know:

- Each medicine's brand and generic name
- Your child's dose
- When and how it is supposed to be given

- When it should be stopped or increased and
- When to refill it

You need to be able to give medicines using the proper device with the proper technique and know how to clean and maintain the device. You also need to teach others who care for your child how to give medicines. The personnel at school or day care may tell you that they know how to give asthma treatments, but it doesn't always mean that they were taught correctly.

In our busy lives, sometimes parents put the responsibility on children to take their own medicine because they seem old enough or smart enough to do it. Talk with your pediatrician about your child's behavior and development in order to determine how ready and able your child is to assume this job independently. As children with any chronic condition grow and develop, they should begin to take on increasing responsibility for their own care. But even so, they will still need supervision and support from their parents.

To be absolutely clear about the medicine plan for your child, you need to communicate with your child's health care professionals and ask whatever questions you may have. Both parents and professionals need to review together whether the medicine is being given correctly—whether the parent is administering the medicine or the child is taking it himself.

SCHEDULING

Correct use of asthma medicines and devices also requires consistent scheduling. In the hectic pace of our lives, monitoring the use of medicine takes some forethought and planning. To keep your child's asthma under control, he needs to take his asthma and allergy medicines regularly. Medicines will help most if they're taken correctly at about the same time every day. Many families find that setting up a regular routine helps them remember to give the medicine to a young child. It also helps older children and teens who can take their own medicine do so without a lot of reminding.

A good time for taking inhaled medicines is in the morning at tooth-brushing time. This way a child can use his inhaler and then brush his teeth. This assures that he takes his medicine and rinses away any residue that might still be in his mouth—and it ensures that he brushes his teeth as well. Sometimes older children like to keep it at their bed-side to take as soon as they wake up and before going to sleep. Encourage your child to find a system that works best for him.

For children who need medicine more than once a day, try to schedule the later doses around something that happens regularly. Some do well with a routine that has them take another dose when they get home from school in the late afternoon. It's easy to remember, and it saves the embarrassment that some feel when they need to use their inhaler or take other medicine in front of their friends and classmates.

Peak flow readings are best taken first thing in the morning and again in the early evening. If your child uses an everyday bronchodilator drug such as salmeterol (Serevent), he should check his peak flow before he takes the medicine.

What are appropriate responsibilities for children in managing their medicines? In general, medicines should be kept out of reach of children until they can understand dangers of taking medicines inappropriately. For most children, this is age ten. Even though we want older children to begin to take responsibility for their medicines, they still need to be monitored by parents. It is recommended that most children be given their medicines by their parents until they are at least eleven years old. Of course, you know your child best and may want to wait until he is even older. After a child has been given this responsibility, parents should still make sure that they check the medicines each month to monitor their appropriate use.

Care of Asthma Devices

Caring for asthma devices is as important as using them in the correct way. In general, these devices require very little care. Peak flow meters can be washed monthly with soapy water.

A spacer is easy to care for if you simply follow the directions that come with it. Most spacers need to be washed with dishwashing soap to remove medicine residue, then rinsed and allowed to air-dry once a week. Whenever you wash your child's spacer, make sure that none of the plastic or rubber, such as the valve or ring where the MDI fits into the spacer, are dried out or cracked. If they are, replace the spacer. Keep the caps on MDI/spacers to keep out any tiny foreign particles that could be inhaled.

Nebulizers have to be cleaned properly. The air compressor should be wiped off with a damp cloth only. The filter needs to be replaced once a month or sooner if it becomes discolored. More filters can be ordered from the durable medical equipment company that provided you with the nebulizer. Nebulizer tubing should be changed each month. The tubing may be disposable or reusable. Tubing with a mouthpiece or mask has to be replaced. A disposable nebulizer should last a month and should be cleaned *after each use*.

Wash the nebulizer with water and dishwashing detergent, rinse it, and disinfect it by soaking it in a solution of water and vinegar. Some reusable nebulizers can be washed in the dishwasher and also need to be disinfected. A reusable nebulizer may last between six months to one year.

STORING MEDICINES AT HOME

It is best if all the asthma medicine is kept together in a plastic container that is stored in a cool, dry place, and out of the reach of younger children. Some preparations of medicine have specific care concerns. Dry powder inhalers, for example, need to be in a moisture-free environment to keep the powder dry. This means that you don't want to keep DPIs in the bathroom medicine cabinet because that room tends to have a lot of moisture from baths and showers. Other areas to avoid include the basement, the top of the refrigerator, or near leaky faucets. If moisture causes the powder to cake, your child will probably not get a full dose of the medicine when he inhales.

Metered dose inhalers and spacers should be stored with the cap on. If not, a small object may be present in the inhaler or spacer that could get stuck in your child's airway when he inhales. Most importantly all medicines should be out of the reach of younger children (under ten years old).

7

Asthma
Day to Day

Will asthma necessarily keep children from climbing on jungle gyms, riding bikes, skateboarding, swimming, dancing, and doing all the other things that youngsters want to do? *No.*

With proper medicine and recognition of symptoms, children with asthma should have no symptoms, no missed school days, and no restrictions on their activities. If you or your child don't quite believe that, take a look at the Olympic gold medalists, professional athletes, Oscar-winning actors, doctors, and even presidents of the United States who have asthma (for example, Charles Dickens, John F. Kennedy, Kristi Yamaguchi, Sharon Stone, and Ricki Lake; see Resources for a long list of famous people with asthma).

A "normal life" with asthma means children should have no coughing, wheezing, shortness of breath, or chest pain during the day or night. They should be able to participate in activities without limitation. Flares should be rare when asthma is properly controlled, as discussed in chapter 4.

Minimal side effects from medicine are another important goal of good asthma care. Children should grow to normal adulthood without any lifelong side effects or disabilities. It's important, therefore, to work with your physician to make sure that your child is on the right medicines. Your mutual goal is for your child to lead a normal life, so proper medicine is necessary to prevent, control, and treat symptoms. The medicines should not be too many or too few.

Identifying triggers that set off symptoms is another essential ingredient in preventing flares and assuring a normal life for children with asthma. These triggers include various allergens such as pet dander, dust, pollen, and viral infections. Some triggers are easier to avoid or eliminate than others. Viral infection is the most common trigger in young children and nearly impossible to avoid. But an annual influenza vaccination (a flu shot) will help prevent asthma flares from the flu virus.

BE PREPARED WITH A PLAN

If your child's physician or nurse practitioner hasn't already helped you make a written asthma management plan, be sure to ask about one at your next appointment. Your child's plan should detail a specific course of action to start whenever symptoms appear. Plans will vary from physician to physician and patient to patient.

An asthma management plan used at The Children's Hospital of Philadelphia is included on pages 220–222 in Resources. You're encouraged to copy it, take it to your child's doctor, and use it as a model to construct your child's individual plan. Whether you use this or any other form, a clearly written asthma management plan should contain the following components that are tailored to your own child:

- A list of everyday controller medicines, with instructions about which medicines to give, how much, and how often;
- Your child's "personal best" reading if he or she uses a peak flow meter;
- Instructions for using an inhaler when breathing becomes troublesome during exercise or sports, how many puffs to take and when to take them (usually fifteen to thirty minutes before exercise);

- Instructions about what to do when symptoms start, which quick-relief medicine to use, how many puffs to inhale and how often, or what medicine to give by nebulizer and how often;
- Instructions about what to do when a flare starts, with a range of peak flow meter readings during a flare;
- Instructions about when to give extra anti-inflammatory medicine, name of the specific medicine, how many days to continue giving it, and number of times per day;
- An emergency section: what to do if symptoms get worse, name and number of physician to call, when to call 911 or go to an emergency room.

An asthma management plan has three levels. Think of it as a ladder. You move up a level or step as symptoms become more serious or frequent. Doctors have developed a color-coded system modeled after a traffic light to represent the three levels of severity:

1. **Green—Go!** The first level is the everyday plan—the daily controller medicines your child takes to keep asthma symptoms away even when she's feeling well.

2. **Yellow—Caution!** Move to the second level when symptoms appear (coughing, wheezing, or chest tightness). This level includes use of the quick-relief medicines (usually albuterol) that your child needs right away to get the symptoms back under control and usually includes increasing the dose of inhaled corticosteroids or adding an oral corticosteroid.

3. **Red—Medical Alert!** The third level is more serious. It is used when symptoms continue or get worse. This part of the asthma management plan helps you decide how much more quick-relief medicine to give and if your child needs to see the doctor or go to the emergency room.

The key to asthma control is finding the right controller medicine. Controller medicines must be taken every day, although for some children they sometimes can be stopped in certain seasons. But don't stop the medicine without first checking with your child's physician or nurse practitioner.

WHEN IS IT NECESSARY TO START EXTRA ASTHMA MEDICINES?

When your child has some coughing, wheezing, or shortness of breath, it is time to give her albuterol, the quick-relief medicine. If she needs to use albuterol more than two times in one day, it is time to move to the next step in the management plan.

When a child has a cold or asthma flare for any other reason (such as coming in contact with a neighbor's pet or visiting a home where a smoker lives), she will also develop more symptoms and need quick-relief medicine.

Whether a child needs quick-relief medicines two times in a day for a cold or any other reason, an asthma flare is starting, and it's time to move to the next step in the management plan—albuterol and extra inhaled corticosteroids.

MONITORING SYMPTOMS AND RECOGNIZING WHEN A FLARE IS STARTING

For asthma control to be ideal, it is important to recognize changes in symptoms. Your careful observations will help determine whether your child's asthma is becoming better or worse. Symptoms vary from child to child and may include coughing, wheezing, shortness of breath, rapid breathing, difficulty catching his breath, chest pain, or increased mucus in the chest. These symptoms may appear alone or in combination with one another.

You can monitor symptoms in two basic ways: by recognizing and tracking symptoms as they appear or by measuring breathing with a peak flow meter. The National Institutes of Health recognizes both methods as accurate. The choice depends on the child, family, and physician or nurse practitioner to determine what is best.

Symptom Recognition

This simply means identifying your child's asthma symptoms and noticing when and how they change. Is he coughing at night? Complaining of chest tightness? Breathing rapidly? Showing decreased tolerance for physical activity? Does he cough anytime he plays or laughs? Is he waking up at night with wheezing? If your child is a toddler, does he start coughing or wheezing after a temper tantrum? Or does your teenager develop shortness of breath when laughing?

You are probably the one who will recognize most symptoms. But if your child is school-age, he might be better able to recognize his own symptoms, like coughing at school or while playing sports. You are more likely to observe symptoms in a toddler, but you might also hear coughing at night in an adolescent.

Many families like to keep a daily diary to track symptoms and medicine use. The diary can be a notebook where a child's symptoms are written down in a table where the symptoms are listed and checked off as they occur. However you design a daily diary, keep it simple. It's helpful to note the date and time of day that symptoms appear in order to notice patterns. Take the diary to your child's medical appointments because your doctor or nurse practitioner will find it useful. A sample diary appears on page 95.

With young children, hints often appear to tip you off that symptoms may be starting. A very young child will not be able to tell you that his chest is tight or he's having shortness of breath. You'll probably notice that your child gets a little cranky or tired, or has a tickle in his throat, several hours or even a day before more noticeable asthma symptoms appear. Learn to recognize your child's early warning signs. If he's old enough to talk, encourage him to tell you if he's not feeling right, even if he can't explain exactly what the problem is.

Peak Flow Meter

A peak flow meter provides a good way to keep tabs on symptoms and airway conditions. This small, handheld device measures how much air

A Typical Diary of Symptoms

Daytime Symptoms

How much of the time did you have trouble breathing today?	None of the time	A little of the time	Some of the time	A good bit of the time	Most of the time	All of the time
How much did your asthma bother you today?	Didn't bother me	Bothered me a little	Bothered me somewhat	Bothered me a good deal	Bothered me very much	Bothered me as much as possible
How much of the time did your asthma limit your physical activity, like running, jumping, sports, bike riding, etc., today?	None of the time	A little of the time	Some of the time	A good bit of the time	Most of the time	All of the time

Nighttime Symptoms

Were you awakened by asthma during the night or in the morning?	No	Once	More than once	Awake all night

a child can breathe out. If her airways are starting to swell and tighten with asthma flare, the peak flow reading will drop. Although the peak flow meter is a valuable tool for asthma management, it is not for everyone. Children younger than age five or six usually can't use it. An adult should supervise the use of a peak flow meter until the child is fourteen to sixteen years old.

Peak flow meters are inexpensive and available without a prescription at any pharmacy. Ask your doctor or nurse practitioner which type is best for your child. To keep the readings consistent, stick with the same brand when you buy a new one. For younger children with smaller lung capacity, you may want to choose a low-range model instead of the regular adult kind.

Young children have lower peak flow readings than older, taller children. Because young children can't blow very hard, their numbers may barely move on an adult type of peak flow model. If they can't see their numbers moving up, young children sometimes feel discouraged about their readings. A low-range meter is not only more accurate and age-appropriate for smaller children, it will also give them more positive reinforcement as they see their numbers rise.

The peak flow meter measures your child's peak expiratory flow rate (PEFR), or how much air flows out of her lungs as she breathes out forcefully. Think of it as a thermometer for the lungs. Just as a thermometer tells you if your child has a fever and how high it is, a peak flow meter tells you if her airways are starting to close down and by how much.

Learning to use the peak flow meter takes a little practice. To get an accurate reading, have your child follow these seven steps:

1. Hold the peak flow meter by the handle and set the pointer to zero. Be sure your child's fingers don't block the pointer or the hole in the back of some meters because this will give an inaccurate reading.
2. Stand up straight.
3. Take a really deep breath and fill the lungs with as much air as they will hold.
4. Put the mouthpiece in the mouth, and breathe out through the mouth as hard and fast as possible. The goal is a *fast blast,* not a

slow blow. Make sure your child doesn't cough or spit into the meter because this will make the reading higher than it really is. Your child needs to give her best effort. If she doesn't breathe in as deep as possible and blow out as hard as possible, the reading will be lower than it should be.

5. Look at the scale on the meter to see where the pointer has stopped. Write down the number.

6. Repeat the process twice and reset the pointer to zero each time. If your child has learned how to use the meter properly, the numbers on the scale from all her tries should be fairly close together. If they're not, she probably needs to practice the technique a bit more.

7. Write down the highest number of all her tries. Don't average all the readings together. The highest number is your child's *personal best peak flow* for that day.

No matter how often you check peak flow readings, keep an ongoing written record of them. A simple piece of paper with the date, time of day, and peak flow reading is all you really need. If you can make a note of any other information about your child's health at the time of the reading, that's even better. If the peak flow reading is low, for example, and your child also has a cold or was visiting a friend with a cat, that information helps explain the reading. Peak flows and any other information you can provide will be very helpful to you and the doctor as a way to determine how well your child's asthma is under control. It will also help you track down asthma triggers and help your child understand why she should avoid them.

Understanding the Peak Flow Numbers

Once a child has mastered the peak flow meter, it's time to find her *personal best* reading. This is the number that will be her benchmark, the one you compare all other readings with in order to see if they're below normal.

To find your child's personal best reading, start on a day when she's feeling well and her asthma is under good control. Take three good readings and find the personal best number in the morning before she takes her everyday controller medicine. Repeat the process each day at the same time for two to three weeks. The best numbers from each reading should be fairly close together. If they are, take the best number over the whole period and use that as your child's personal best.

As your child grows, her personal best peak flow number should rise along with her increasing lung size. Redo the personal best readings every six months or whenever your physician or nurse practitioner recommends it to keep the number accurate and in tune with her growing size.

Every peak flow meter comes with a table that tells the normal values for that meter. In other words, the table lists what a normal reading on that particular brand of peak flow meter should be for an imaginary average child of your child's height. Don't worry if your child's personal best peak flow isn't the same as the average given by the meter manufacturer or in the table on the following page.

Green, Yellow, Red Zones

Doctors have used these readings to develop a color-coded peak flow zone system modeled after a traffic light similar to the one for symptom recognition (see page 92). Here's how it works:

- **Green zone—Go!** Your child is taking everyday controller medicine and doing well, with no cough, wheeze, shortness of breath, or chest tightness. He sleeps through the night and his activity is normal. His peak flow meter reading is 80 percent or more of his personal best.

- **Yellow zone—Caution!** Your child's asthma is getting worse, even though he's been taking his everyday medicine. His airways are starting to narrow. He's coughing, wheezing, and short of breath; asthma symptoms are waking him up at night; and he's not as active as usual. An asthma flare might be starting. His peak flow meter reading is 50 percent to 80 percent of his personal best.

- **Red zone—Medical alert!** The quick-relief medicine isn't helping, or the asthma is getting worse. Your child is having an asthma flare. He's very short of breath, wheezing and coughing a lot, and his peak flow meter reading is 50 percent or less of his personal best.

Average Peak Flow Readings for Children

Child's Height (inches)	Green Zone (average peak flow)	Yellow Zone (50%–80% average)	Red Zone (less than 50% average)
43	147	74–118	less than 74
44	160	80–128	less than 80
45	173	87–139	less than 87
46	187	94–150	less than 94
47	200	100–160	less than 100
48	214	107–171	less than 107
49	227	114–182	less than 114
50	240	120–192	less than 120
51	254	127–203	less than 127
52	267	134–214	less than 134
53	280	140–224	less than 140
54	293	147–234	less than 147
55	307	154–246	less than 154
56	320	160–256	less than 160
57	334	167–267	less than 167
58	347	174–278	less than 174
59	360	180–288	less than 180
60	373	187–298	less than 187
61	387	194–310	less than 194
62	400	200–320	less than 200
63	413	207–330	less than 207
64	427	214–342	less than 214
65	440	220–352	less than 220
66	454	227–363	less than 227

WHICH SYSTEM IS BETTER FOR YOUR CHILD, SYMPTOM RECOGNITION OR PEAK FLOW?

Every child is different, and the choice of a system will depend on your individual child. Let's look at how two children, Tyrone and Tammy, learned to gain control of their asthma by these two systems.

Tyrone, twelve, has had asthma for six years. His asthma symptoms used to appear anytime he caught a cold, especially in the first few days, when he'd wake at night, coughing and wheezing. As his cold improved, his night symptoms disappeared, but the cough hung on for about ten days.

His doctor had given Tyrone a quick-relief (albuterol) inhaler with a spacer to use whenever he had a cold. That solution had worked well—until recently. Tyrone began to need his inhaler even when he didn't have a cold. He used it when playing basketball because he got short of breath and started coughing five minutes into a game.

After three months of increasing symptoms, he went back to his doctor. Tyrone's lung function tests had decreased. His peak flow meter reading was 68 percent of his personal best. His doctor started Tyrone on inhaled corticosteroids, gave him an asthma management plan, and told him to begin the plan whenever his symptoms start to change: for example, when he needs albuterol twice in one day, and again when he feels short of breath.

At a follow-up appointment three months later, Tyrone reported that he could play basketball without problems. But when he caught a cold, the wheezing and coughing made him miss two weeks of school. When the doctor asked if he was following his management plan, Tyrone said he started it after he'd had the cold for two or three days.

That was the problem. His physician explained: "You need to begin your management plan as soon as you start waking up at night with wheezing or coughing, or when you need to use your albuterol two times in one day, because those are signs your asthma is starting to flare." Tyrone agreed and added that he could usually tell when his asthma was about to get worse because he'd feel a tightness in his chest the day beforehand. By his next follow-up visit, Tyrone had absorbed the lesson. He'd had one cold but started his management plan immediately and didn't miss any school.

What can we learn from Tyrone? This young man has good symptom recognition. He can spot early signs of a flare and recognize when his asthma is getting worse. And he learned to use his management plan to enable him to control his asthma.

Let's look at another child, ten-year-old Tammy:

Tammy had been feeling well, with no apparent symptoms, when she suddenly couldn't breathe. Her father rushed her to the nearest ER. A week later, she had a follow-up appointment with her pediatrician, who also happened to be Tyrone's doctor. Tammy reported that she has no problem playing soccer. She is her team's goalie and never coughs or wheezes at games. When the doctor asked why she played goalie, Tammy said she got out of breath faster than her teammates so the coach made her goalie.

The doctor started Tammy on inhaled steroids and gave her the same management plan as Tyrone's. On a three-month follow-up visit, Tammy excitedly told the doctor that she could now keep up with her teammates on the field, had switched positions to offense, and scored her first goal. But Tammy and her mother were confused about something. A month ago, Tammy again got sick suddenly and went to the emergency room. Her spirometry was improved but not to the normal range.

Her doctor asked about her medicine use. Tammy had been taking her daily medicines but hadn't started her management plan at any time during the last three months. So the doctor taught her how to use a peak flow meter. Green, yellow, and red zones were set based on her personal best and her spirometry.

A few months later, Tammy told the doctor that she was doing fine—no problems in sports and no sudden asthma flares that sent her to the ER. Her peak flow readings were all above 230, except for one week when they dropped into the yellow zone. Then she started her management plan and her peak flows returned to the green zone within five days. Interestingly, Tammy didn't notice any difference in symptoms during that time.

What can we learn from Tammy? Some children have flares without obvious symptoms. Peak flow meters are perfect for youngsters like Tammy. Many people recognize symptoms before changes in their peak flow readings, while others see a drop in peak flows before they notice any symptoms. Tyrone's and Tammy's experiences represent two typical situations: either symptom recognition or a peak flow meter will work for different children. You and your doctor will decide which way works best for your individual child.

THE CHALLENGE: REMEMBERING TO TAKE DAILY MEDICINES

A big part of keeping asthma under control and preventing flares is to make sure your child takes everyday medicines regularly—even when feeling well. This isn't easy, but it is critically important to managing asthma. Nobody likes to take medicine every day. People remember to take medicine when they are sick because they want to feel better. But it's normal for children, as well as adults, to overlook daily medicine when they feel fine.

Parents can take several steps to make taking asthma medicines a normal part of life and not a daily battle.

- **Explain why the medicine is needed.** Because children and adults feel the benefits of quick-relief medicines right away, they immediately understand why they need them. Taking everyday medicines to prevent symptoms is a bigger challenge. Explain, in language your child will understand, that this medicine keeps asthma away just like daily toothbrushing keeps cavities away.

- **Be firm and matter-of-fact without nagging.** Once your child understands that taking the daily medicine is simply the way it is—it's not negotiable or optional—he'll accept the situation. And you can always say, "The doctor said . . . ."

- **Set a routine.** Many parents find that setting up a regular routine helps their child remember to take the medicine every day at the same time. If your child uses inhaled steroids, for example, a good time to take the medicine would be right before he brushes his teeth in the morning and at night. This helps him take the medicine regularly, and it also makes sure he rinses out his mouth after using it. For any once-a-day medicine, set a time to take the medicine, such as at breakfast or dinner.

When your child first starts to take everyday asthma medicines, you and he probably won't notice much improvement right away. Improvement happens gradually, usually over several weeks. After a couple of months on the medicine, your child should have fewer or no asthma symptoms. At this point, help him look back over the past couple of months. When you count up all the nights he slept straight through and the days he went to school and played normally, you'll both realize that the everyday medicines really are helping. That should do a lot to help everyone stick with the medicine routine.

8

Managing an Asthma Flare

One of the characteristics of asthma is that it changes over time, sometimes unexpectedly. Every child with asthma has some episodes of increased symptoms. The overall pattern of symptoms—how consistently she is at her best and how often flares occur—will determine the type of treatment plan prescribed.

Children with persistent or daily symptoms and those with frequent flares need daily controller medicines. But all children with asthma, even those who don't take daily medicines, need a plan to manage flares. To use the plan properly, the family and child must know when to start it. New flares can begin at any time and in unpredictable ways. But all new flares can be recognized at their very beginning.

As a parent, you can best help your child through a flare by being prepared and staying calm. Use your child's asthma management plan and your own understanding of your child to give him the appropriate medicines right away and get her to her doctor or an emergency room if necessary. A major reason children with asthma end up in the hospital is because a flare has gone on for too long. Learn to recognize the warning signs of a flare and act immediately to treat them.

Caryn is an active seven-year-old with ten-year-old twin brothers. She always seems to be in motion—dancing to CDs, taking ballet lessons, running around outside with her neighborhood friends. Since Caryn's asthma was diagnosed two years ago, her parents have seen that she takes her controller medicine twice a day. She very rarely has asthma symptoms, but when they do appear she uses her albuterol inhaler for quick relief.

Caryn caught a cold in early January. Her nose ran, she sneezed and coughed occasionally, but her parents didn't think it necessary to keep her home from school. Caryn seemed otherwise normal— she teased her brothers, ran away from them when they dished it back, and occasionally got into a fairly friendly wrestling match with one or both of them.

A few days into the cold, Caryn's parents heard her coughing more often, especially after laughing with her brothers. And she seemed more tired than usual. Instead of actively playing, she lolled on the sofa and watched TV. Caryn's parents heard her coughing in the middle of the night, but she didn't wake up. When they heard the coughing, they assumed it was another symptom of her cold, that it had moved from her head to her chest and was per-haps bronchitis. "Maybe we should call the pediatrician tomor-row," they thought.

RECOGNIZING THE START
OF AN ASTHMA FLARE

A basic definition of a flare is any worsening of asthma symptoms. In the simplest terms, mild increases in symptoms need less medicine than severe or prolonged symptoms. In general, if your child needs more than one dose of albuterol or quick-relief medicine in a day, a new flare may be starting. A sure sign that a flare has started is when symptoms such as night cough (after midnight) are present. As discussed in chapter 7, the family and child can use either "symptom recognition" or peak flow monitoring to detect the beginning of a new flare. Each is effective, but symptom recognition is most commonly used. Whether mild or severe, worsening symptoms means that inflammation is increasing in the lungs. The more rapidly symptoms rise or the more severe they become, the greater the increase in inflammation. Therefore, for any level of severity, increased doses of anti-inflammatory or controller medicine should be given.

Detecting a new flare is easy in a child who is under good control and has no daily symptoms and normal lung function. The start of symptoms such as cough, wheezing, shortness of breath, chest pain or tightness usually tells us that control is slipping and a flare may be starting. Another sign may be your child's decreased activity or need for quick-relief medicine such as albuterol.

Many parents find it helpful to think about their child's previous flares in order to identify which symptoms indicate that a flare is beginning. For example, have past flares usually been triggered by a cold virus? The trigger may not be a single symptom; it's also important to know what *mixture* of symptoms your child commonly has in a flare. Most children cough a lot when asthma worsens. This is hard to miss. Some children only cough a little at the start of a flare, unless their flare is severe. For these children, flares may be characterized by shortness of breath, chest pain, wheezing, or decreased activity. Children with less obvious symptoms may get worse without their parents noticing, unless they have learned to recognize the typical pattern of symptoms for their child.

Some children may wheeze infrequently or rarely. In these youngsters, obviously, wheezing cannot be used to detect a flare. But most children will have a mixture of symptoms including cough, shortness of breath, chest pain or tightness, wheeze and/or fatigue. And parents can learn to remember this typical "snapshot" of their child when she has worsening symptoms. It is very helpful for parents to discuss this picture with their child's asthma caregiver. In this way, everyone will learn more about the child's asthma, and symptom recognition will get better and better over time.

Parents should also remember how their child tends to handle her symptoms. Most children cannot hold back their symptoms, but some will attempt to hide them because they want to please their parents or not make them worry. A child who conceals or denies symptoms can delay the detection of a new flare unless peak flows are monitored on a regular basis. Obviously, other circumstances can interfere with recognition of symptoms, such as separation of parent and child during work or school hours.

ONGOING SYMPTOMS

It's important to consider how a flare unfolds. At the very beginning, symptoms may appear to be very mild and remain so for a day or two before more serious problems appear. Typically, peak flow rates will begin to drop at the same time that symptoms increase. Sometimes the very first sign that a flare might begin is the appearance of a common cold or upper respiratory tract symptoms, such as runny nose, nasal congestion, or fever. Be aware, however, that not every cold virus will trigger an asthma flare. Also remember that as a child gets older, cold symptoms can be very mild or absent, even though a virus has infected the respiratory tract and will trigger a new asthma flare. In this case, the presence of nasal symptoms is not a useful clue.

When an asthma flare becomes severe, virtually all children will have either a cough or other lung-specific symptoms (such as wheezing) late at night—usually after midnight. These nighttime symptoms can last for one or two nights in milder flares or much longer with severe flares. And as a new flare begins to get better, coughing and other symptoms during this midnight-to-6-A.M. time frame begin to disappear. This decrease should reassure you that a flare is changing for the better, and the medicine plan is working. If symptoms don't improve during this time frame, look at your plan again. More medicine and perhaps monitoring may be indicated, so let your doctor or nurse practitioner know of your concern.

Parents and children are often confused and frightened when symptoms reach their fullest expression late at night. Why do symptoms get worse after midnight or in the early morning hours? An asthma flare represents increased inflammation in the lungs. During the late-night hours, protective mechanisms against inflammation decrease. Blood levels of cortisol and adrenaline decrease during this time, allowing inflammation to increase.

Another reason that symptoms flare is the tendency of the lungs' airways to be "twitchy" or tighten easily. This is called "airway hyper-reactivity." Simple things like laughing or crying hard, running and playing or breathing cold air make a child cough, get short of breath, wheeze, or have chest tightness or pain. If there is enough closure of the airway, this obstruction causes more severe shortness of breath.

This "twitchiness" is the first symptom to appear with a new flare and the last to leave. In fact, with any asthma flare, an increase in lung twitchiness can last for days or even weeks. A child who is completely well between cold virus–triggered flares might have the tendency to cough easily for a prolonged time after a flare. After nighttime cough is gone, the child usually begins an increase in daytime activity like playing outside. When he comes in for dinner, he might cough all evening before midnight. It might seem that a new flare is starting, but after midnight there are no symptoms. In this common situation, a child needs only some quick-relief medicine before bedtime. If no new symptoms occur after midnight, a new flare is *not* beginning. This youngster only has a temporary increase in "twitchiness" from his last flare.

Increased production of mucus by the lungs is another reason that symptoms occur during asthma flares. This happens at the beginning of a flare, but the excess mucus will not flow up the bronchial tree very well until the severe tightening of the airways begins to decrease. When the flare is at its height, a child may cough as though he wants to get something out of his chest, but nothing may come up. Later when the airways are more open, or after a bronchodilator treatment opens them farther, mucus begins to travel upward more easily. This may cause cough in itself. Thick mucus secretions need forceful coughs to move upward through narrow passageways. Often a treatment with albuterol or other bronchodilator may increase the cough because lung secretions are loosened. This is to be expected and should not be a cause for alarm unless the cough and choking is not relieved within a brief period of time.

After night coughing diminishes, airways are typically more open, and coughs caused by "loose" secretions of mucus become more promi-nent. Coughing usually occurs upon waking in the morning, and a "loose" cough appears during the day. This pattern should not be con-fused with mucus made in the nose or postnasal drip because the lungs make their own mucus. Typically, the period of time when a child shows symptoms from increased airway mucus will end before the extra twitchiness does.

At best, no signs such as nighttime cough or increased mucus should be present between flares. If symptoms begin and quick-relief medicines are needed, a new flare likely has begun, and your management plan should be started. Remember that any child who has daily symptoms of severe persistent asthma will have trouble detecting the start of a new flare. These children have most symptoms on a daily basis, including night cough. Their symptoms don't turn on and off, and therefore these children have significant difficulty knowing when to begin their manage-ment plans. For these youngsters to successfully manage their asthma, daily symptoms (especially the nighttime symptoms) need to be reduced by adjusting daily controller medicines and environmental controls.

When Caryn woke up the next morning, she seemed a little better. She said she felt fine and was eager to go to school because her class was having a special art program that afternoon. Caryn only coughed once or twice during breakfast, so her parents—needing to rush to work themselves—sent her off to meet the school bus and forgot about calling the pediatrician. That night Caryn woke up coughing hard at four o'clock. She went to her parents' room and told them she was having a lot of trouble breathing. The scared look on her face alarmed her parents. They dialed the pediatrician's number, got the answering service, and explained that they thought this could be an emergency.

When the doctor called back a few minutes later, she asked Caryn's mother about the symptoms—what they were, how long they'd lasted—and asked if Caryn had begun her asthma manage-ment plan for flares. Her mother immediately realized that she hadn't even thought "asthma." She'd been assuming all along that this was "just a cold."

The pediatrician told her to give Caryn albuterol immediately for quick relief and to increase the dose of Flovent, the inhaled corticosteroid specified in Caryn's asthma management plan, and to continue using this anti-inflammatory medicine for the next five to seven days.

The pediatrician called back a few days later to see how Caryn was doing. The albuterol had helped, she'd started the increased dose of Flovent, but she still had some nighttime coughing for two more nights, so her parents had decided to keep her home from school for two days.

The doctor reminded her mother that Caryn was close to needing a course of oral steroids and told her to review Caryn's asthma management plan and immediately take action when symptoms arise or change in the future. Caryn's mother said she was embarrassed that she hadn't linked her daughter's recent symptoms to asthma.

"It's easy to overlook," the doctor replied, "because Caryn's asthma has been under good control for months. But the key is to recognize symptoms quickly and notice any changes in symptom patterns because they can signal the beginning of a flare. Even symptoms of a cold can be asthma triggers, and you want to take control sooner rather than later."

TREATING A FLARE

It's helpful to review the management plan for the flares section of the sample asthma management action plan (pages 220–222). The initial treatment for a new flare is recommended to include three components:

1. Bronchodilator therapy to relieve symptoms of obstruction.
2. Increased doses of controller or anti-inflammatory medicine (corticosteroid) for a defined period—typically five to seven days.
3. Continuation of other controller medicines for asthma whose doses are not adjusted during new flares.

As discussed in previous chapters, bronchodilators help open airways narrowed by bronchospasm, swelling, and increased secretions of mucus. Usually higher doses are used during a flare than are used for mild symptom relief or pretreatment before exercise. Because your child may have difficulty taking a deep breath or holding her breath during a flare, a mist of bronchodilator delivered by a nebulizer may be more effective. However, equally effective doses of bronchodilator can be delivered by metered dose inhaler (MDI) and spacer, provided the dose is adequate. Your child's management plan should prescribe appropriate doses of quick-relief medicine. The bronchodilator can be used up to every four hours at home, but when this fails to control symptoms, call your physician or asthma specialist.

Many asthma caregivers recommend starting extra anti-inflammatory medicines at this point. If a flare truly seems to have begun, increased doses of inhaled or oral corticosteroids should be used at this point to treat inflammation. Follow your child's management plan and don't wait to start the corticosteroids. Delaying may diminish their effectiveness, since inflammation levels can continue to rise without them.

The first option for corticosteroids to treat flares is an inhaled form delivered either by metered dose inhaler with a spacer or by a nebulizer. Both are effective if the doses are adequate and the devices are used properly. As a general rule of thumb, either a tripled or doubled dose of the established, effective daily controller dose of inhaled steroids will do the trick. For example, if your child was receiving 100 mcg of an inhaled corticosteroid twice daily, an action plan might increase it to 200 mcg either twice or three times per day for one week. It is helpful to give the bronchodilator before the inhaled steroid to enhance delivery deep into the lungs.

The use of inhaled steroids for a flare, instead of oral steroids, is an effective way to decrease steroid exposure for a child. Because the inhaled form goes directly into the lungs, much smaller amounts are needed than with oral steroids. If a child fails to improve after two or three days, and especially if night coughing gets worse, oral steroids may be recommended. Using oral steroids is highly effective to treat an asthma flare, but some families are reluctant to start them unless a child is quite ill. Most physicians agree, but when inhaled steroids fail to stop the flare, oral steroids are usually effective and can prevent the need for emergency room care or hospitalization. Some doctors may recommend using oral corticosteroids at the beginning of a flare in children whose asthma is more severe or whose peak flow rate has decreased. The pros and cons of the use of inhaled versus oral corticosteroids for flares should be discussed with you child's doctor.

When you start a management plan for a suspected flare and it's clear within twenty-four hours that all symptoms are gone, there's no need for quick-relief albuterol. All flares should be treated with the management plan, including increased doses of inhaled steroids, unless the flare is very mild and includes no night cough in a child whose asthma is well controlled.

Unfortunately, the timing of new flares is unpredictable. Some children may have several flares in a row. If one flare follows on the heels of another, the second will be typically worse in intensity and/or duration. But the new flare will be more easily controlled if the preceding flare was effectively managed. Families who've watched repeated flares spin out of control quickly understand the advantage of treating early flares adequately. It becomes much easier and more intuitive each time.

Every management plan should provide names and numbers of physicians (primary doctor, nurse practitioner, or asthma specialist) to call if the management plan begun at home fails to provide control. A simple guide is that if a quick-relief medicine is needed more than every four hours, or if severe symptoms are apparent, treatment at home should end, and the child should be taken to an emergency room as soon as possible.

WHEN IT'S OVER

Once night coughing has stopped, sleep returns, and asthma symptoms are well controlled by using albuterol less than every four hours, you can consider sending your child back to school or day care. You may need to wait longer before she can engage in full physical activity without symptoms, although preexercise bronchodilators may be useful. You should consult with your doctor with each flare.

Good asthma control means no symptoms at the child's best normal lung function and the fewest, mildest flares possible. Good control of day-to-day asthma symptoms will provide a reduction in the number and severity of flares. Each child must have a management plan for flares and become an expert in its use. Everyone at home, in school, and on the medical care team should understand and have access to the management plan. Every family wants their child to receive the least amount of steroids, but these effective medicines are indicated for use in most flares. All families want to achieve the most control possible over asthma. A management plan that includes appropriate controller and quick-relief medicines, as well as environmental control measures, will allow you to reach this goal.

Caryn's first frightening experience of waking up at 4 A.M. with bad coughing and shortness of breath was never repeated. Her parents learned to recognize the first signs of a flare and immediately referred to the recommendations in her asthma management plan. Later that winter, she started to experience some asthma symptoms, especially after playing outside in cold, dry air and again when she caught another cold. But this time, she used albuterol for quick relief and her parents made sure that she got an increased dose of Flovent for several days to keep airway inflammation under control. Over the next few years, Caryn's occasional flares occurred less frequently, and when they did appear, the symptoms were less intense and didn't escalate or last as long because she and her parents had become more aware and they swung into her action plan right away.

9

Asthma Emergencies

Since three-year-old Robert was diagnosed with asthma a year ago, his symptoms and flares have been minor and easily treated with albuterol. But late one evening, as they were putting him to bed, his parents noticed a change in his breathing. Something was "just different." He seemed to be working harder to breathe. Robert had come down with a cold earlier in the week, and his chronic cough grew worse. When his dad went to check on him at 2 A.M., Robert was sitting up straight, and the muscles in his neck and chest were moving visibly with each breath. He was able to get out only a few words at a time. While Dad gave him an albuterol treatment, his mother counted his breathing rate at forty times per minute. Dad called the family doctor who recommended going immediately to the emergency room.

Most of this book has focused on the importance of controlling asthma-related symptoms that affect your child on a day-to-day basis. That focus is appropriate because asthma is a chronic illness, and the long-term effect of these symptoms may have a profound impact on a child's quality of life at home and school. This chapter, however, will examine a much more dramatic face of the disease—the asthma emergency that every parent fears—as we follow Robert through his trip to the emergency room.

Symptom flares can occur in any child with asthma and, if not managed successfully, can result in an unexpected trip to an emergency department. This chapter addresses how to recognize and manage severe flares of asthma and gives an overview of emergency and hospital care. If you understand this information in advance and review it from time to time, any emergency can be handled more successfully and with less distress for you and your child.

WHO IS AT RISK FOR ASTHMA EMERGENCIES?

Emergency visits, hospitalizations, and even deaths from asthma have all increased over recent decades, and the causes are not entirely clear. A major driving force is certainly the increase in overall asthma rates, which more than doubled from about 3 percent of American children in the 1980s to 7 percent today. But other factors also come into play: children from low socioeconomic backgrounds are more likely to be hospitalized for asthma, possibly reflecting a lack of access to optimal medical care. Signs of poor asthma control, such as past severe flares and frequent albuterol use, have been linked to an increased risk of death from asthma.

The link between poor control and poor outcome suggests some good news about reducing the risk. Studies have shown marked reductions in emergency visits, hospitalizations, and mortality rates when asthma is brought under control with effective treatment. During the 1990s, great effort was devoted to developing new therapies and improving standards of care for asthma. These attempts appear to have had some success, as the most recent statistics show a leveling off in asthma hospitalizations nationwide.

When a child's asthma is under good control and the child is otherwise healthy, there's no need for anxiety about an emergency lurking around the next corner. Children with asthma should be able to travel, go camping, and do all of the other things that are a normal part of growing up. With an appropriate management plan, most asthma flares can be managed without a visit to a hospital. When troubles arise, however, a healthy respect for asthma is appropriate. An important part of any plan is a recognition that *things may not go as expected*, so rapid, immediate care may be necessary.

WHEN IS ASTHMA AN EMERGENCY?

Warning signs of a severe asthma flare vary for individual children. As you know, flares occur when a trigger increases inflammation in the airways of the lung. Research suggests that common colds and flu viruses trigger the great majority of severe flares, although conditions in the environment (such as smoke and allergens) can also be important triggers. Airway inflammation leads to increased mucus production and contraction of the muscles in the airway wall (bronchospasm). When the airways in the lung narrow, more work is needed to push out waste gases, such as carbon dioxide. The body's normal response to this airway obstruction is to increase its effort to breathe by using muscles between the ribs and in the neck, which may become more noticeable than usual, as Robert's parents observed in the middle of the night.

The chest and belly may move in opposite directions like a seesaw as muscles below the diaphragm help to move air up and out of the lungs. A child may stop doing other activities and sit up straight to focus on breathing. His rate of breathing will increase. He may become short of breath and able to speak only a few words at a time. Normal breathing rates vary by age and are displayed on the next page.

Signs like these indicate an important change in the child's condition and require immediate treatment with a quick-relief medicine such as albuterol. If these signs continue, it's time to begin the flare part of your management plan and call your doctor or nurse practitioner. If symptoms get worse despite this treatment, go to an emergency department.

Normal Rates of Breathing While Awake by Age

Age	Normal Rate of Breathing
Less than 2 months	Less than 60 breaths per minute
2–12 months	Less than 50 breaths per minute
1–5 years	Less than 40 breaths per minute
6–8 years	Less than 30 breaths per minute

With most children, particularly infants and toddlers, you can easily observe signs of severe airway obstruction. But other problems can occasionally mimic an asthma flare. In young infants, for example, a nose blocked with mucus can mimic wheezing. Clearing the nose with a suction bulb should resolve the breathing trouble. On the other hand, some children adjust to chronic obstruction of their airways and show few signs even when their condition becomes worse. This usually happens in children with a long history of poorly controlled asthma. For these children, obtaining an objective measurement of lung function by using a peak flow meter can be very helpful. A reduction in peak flow to less than 80 percent of a child's usual best measurement indicates moderate obstruction that should be treated with a quick-relief medicine such as albuterol. A reduction in peak flow to 50 percent of the child's usual best should be considered a severe obstruction that requires immediate evaluation.

WHAT IS THE FIRST STEP IN AN EMERGENCY?

If you recognize the signs of a severe flare *early* there should be enough time to give a quick-relief treatment, call your physician, and get to an emergency department. Most asthma flares have a progression of symptoms over the course of hours, and traveling by ambulance should be unnecessary.

Rarely, a child may develop *sudden* severe symptoms. This type of flare has been associated with risk of death from asthma. In any situation where symptoms seem very severe, activating emergency medical services by calling 911 is appropriate. The time required to travel to a hospital through traffic may be difficult to predict. If your child becomes severely ill in the back of a car, it may be very difficult for you to give appropriate treatment and get help. Ambulances are able to provide albuterol treatments by nebulizer as well as oxygen and other support. Another medicine that ambulance staff may give is epinephrine, an injectable medicine that once was a routine treatment for asthma. An injection of epinephrine may help to open up the airways and allow inhaled medicines to penetrate the lungs better.

Ambulances are typically required to go to the nearest hospital, where more definitive care can be provided. At your next regular office visit, discuss with your pediatrician or nurse practitioner which hospital to choose if an emergency situation should arise. Some physicians have arrangements and admitting privileges at specific hospitals where you'll want to go in an emergency to ensure that your doctor is involved in your child's care.

All hospital emergency departments should be able to provide basic treatment for asthma. In today's competitive health care market, however, many community hospitals have cut back inpatient pediatric units, and these services may not be available. If that is the case and hospitalization is needed, transport to a larger center or children's hospital will be required. Intensive care units (ICUs) for children are even more scarce and are typically located only in large regional centers. Although treatment of asthma in adults and children is similar overall, children's hospitals may offer a more child-centered focus, including child-oriented teaching materials and access to special personnel who help children cope with medical procedures.

BEING PREPARED

Before an emergency arises, it's useful to have on hand a list of things to take with you to an emergency department (see the next page). It's most important to take a copy of your child's asthma management plan so the staff knows what your regular physician has prescribed. Take your child's medicines and devices so that staff can determine that everything is functioning correctly. Peak flow records, if available, can provide information about the current flare and your child's lung function when he's well. Take a favorite toy or other security object to help your child pass the time, and plan that you may need to spend the night in the hospital.

Things to bring to the emergency room:

- Asthma management plan
- Asthma medicines
- Asthma devices (spacer, nebulizer)
- Peak flow records
- Toy or book for your child
- Overnight needs (toiletries, clothes, etc.)

When Robert and his parents arrived at triage (the first section of an emergency department), an ER nurse listened to Robert with a stethoscope. She used a special clip on his finger to determine his oxygen level, which measured 90 percent. The nurse then took Robert back to a room and began the first of several nebulizer treatments. She also gave him a small amount of a liquid steroid medicine by mouth. After several hours, Robert was better but still seemed a bit short of breath. His oxygen level continued to measure 90 percent. The physician discussed the situation with his parents and recommended admitting Robert to the hospital for additional treatments and oxygen.

WHAT TO EXPECT IN THE EMERGENCY DEPARTMENT

Emergency department care usually begins with an assessment at triage to determine the level of illness. For asthma, this includes vital signs (temperature, pulse and breathing rates, and blood pressure) and pulse oximetry, a small clip that attaches to a child's finger or toe to measure the oxygen content of the blood. This device can be frightening to young children, but it does not cause pain. The triage nurse will listen to a child's chest to assess air movement and wheezing. This information will be combined into an overall assessment that is used to decide which patients need immediate care.

Assessment of asthma is subjective, and not all staff members may be familiar or comfortable with assessing young children. It is important to communicate your concerns about your child clearly to the triage nurse, but also recognize that nurses may be trying to treat a number of patients at once. Unfortunately, asthma flares tend to be seasonal and many asthmatic children may come in at the same time, taxing the resources of the hospital. Children with low pulse oximetry usually are brought back immediately to receive oxygen. The oximetry level at which oxygen is required varies by altitude, but it will definitely be required if it is below 90 percent. (Normal is 95 percent or greater.) Low oxygen levels typically are caused by mucus plugging the airways, leading to temporary collapse of areas of the lung (referred to as *atelectasis*). These areas will reexpand as mucus and airway obstruction improves.

Next, a physician, nurse practitioner, or other medical professional will evaluate your child. It is important to relate your child's asthma history and response to treatment for past flares. Some children respond rapidly to treatment, while others take more time. Your child's individual past experience may help the staff to plan for hospitalization or discharge.

Asthma flares in the emergency department are treated by using a combination of medicines that are inhaled and/or systemic (that is, given orally, intravenously, or as a shot). Inhaled treatments typically contain albuterol and other medicines that relax the muscles of the airway. These may be given by an inhaler or by nebulizer.

Typically, much higher and more frequent doses are given in the emergency room than are given at home. This is possible because your child is being monitored closely for side effects, such as a fast heart rate. Your child may feel jittery from the albuterol.

Steroid medicines in the emergency room are typically given by mouth in the form of prednisone or other preparations. Steroid medicines act to reduce inflammation in the lungs and have been shown to improve symptoms of a severe flare within two to four hours. Steroids may also be given in an injectable form, although research has not shown that medicine given by injection provides any clear benefit over medicines taken orally. But oral steroid preparations typically have a bitter taste and may cause vomiting. Newer forms are available (Orapred is an example) that taste better. Oral steroids can also cause temporary hyperactivity in some children and can irritate the stomach, but in general they are safe and effective for short periods of time to treat an asthma flare.

After the initial medicines are given, a child is usually observed for several hours to see how well she responds. This can be frustrating, but it's necessary because the doses of albuterol given initially are higher than home doses, and your child's condition may become worse as the effect decreases. If the response is good, your child will probably be discharged to go home with albuterol to use as needed and a short course of oral prednisone or another steroid.

After returning home, you should continue any regular asthma medicines and call your regular physician for an appointment. The fact that your child needed an emergency room visit suggests that it's time to reexamine the management plan and consider whether changes are needed.

HOSPITALIZATION FOR ASTHMA

If your child doesn't respond well to treatment in the emergency department, the staff will arrange for admission to the hospital. In the past, this typically involved moving to a room upstairs in the hospital where care is supervised by your pediatrician or another physician. Today some hospitals offer other options, such as "overnight" units that are attached to the emergency room and designed for short hospital stays.

Hospital treatment for asthma includes regular treatments with albuterol or another quick-relief medicine. These will be given close together initially and then gradually spaced to see if your child is able to move to a frequency that could be given at home. Again, don't be surprised if the doses given in the hospital are higher than what your doctor usually prescribes. Steroid medicines also are an important part of hospital treatment to reduce inflammation in the airways. Oxygen may be given if needed.

If your child is hospitalized for an asthma emergency, she will undoubtedly meet a number of new people. Nurse practitioners and physician assistants are taking on many of the day-to-day responsibilities of physicians. Respiratory therapists have specific training in asthma and lung diseases and provide inhaled medicines as well as other care. In many hospitals, respiratory therapists have an increasingly important role in assessing patients and teaching families about asthma and the use of medicines. Social workers and case managers may also be involved to plan appropriate services and asthma equipment for your child at discharge. A well-planned team approach has been shown to be the most effective way to take care of asthma in the hospital, and the contribution of each of these health professionals is highly important. And because there's a lot of time available during any hospitalization, this is a good opportunity to ask the staff any questions and review your child's management plan.

IN THE ICU

Occasionally, a child may respond poorly to treatment and require admission to an intensive care unit. Asthma care in the ICU may include continuous albuterol treatments and intravenous medicines. Children with severe obstruction of their airways are unable to eliminate waste gases like carbon dioxide from the lungs. If these gases build up in the bloodstream, they'll cause a child to become sleepy. As a tired child spends less energy on breathing, the waste gas levels can continue to increase until breathing stops altogether. In these situations, insertion of a breathing tube (intubation) is needed, and the child will be placed on a ventilator. The use of a ventilator is difficult and has many potential complications. Fortunately, the need for this type of treatment is rare as new treatments for asthma have become available.

By the end of the next day, Robert was feeling much better. It had been over four hours since his last breathing treatment, and he was out in the playroom with the other children. After a discussion with a nurse practitioner on the asthma unit, Robert's parents realized that his lingering cough was a symptom of asthma. They learned that persistent symptoms, like the cough, can be controlled and prevented. The nurse practitioner also spoke with their family doctor, and they decided to prescribe a daily inhaled steroid. A follow-up appointment was scheduled for later in the week to go over the use of the new medicine. With all this new information in hand, Robert's parents felt much better prepared to take control of his asthma in the future.

RECOVERING FROM AN ASTHMA EMERGENCY

Planning for discharge should begin early in the hospitalization process. Your child's regular physician or nurse practitioner should be involved and a follow-up visit scheduled soon after discharge. The need for hospitalization suggests that your child's management plan needs to be reassessed. Steroid medicines given by mouth will usually be continued for several days after discharge, and albuterol can be given as needed, usually up to a frequency of a dose every four hours. Your child should continue any controller medicines during this period.

While recovering from a severe asthma flare, it is particularly important to be sure your child avoids asthma triggers like smoke because her airways are inflamed and sensitive. During the days following a severe flare, it is appropriate to rest and avoid physical activity although this should be just for a brief period. You and your doctor should discuss when your child is able to return to school or day care.

To summarize, asthma emergencies should generally be preventable by achieving good asthma control with an effective management plan. But even the best efforts sometimes fail and an emergency visit is necessary.

Key points in managing severe flares include:

- Early recognition of symptoms
- Contacting your regular physician
- Seeking care in an appropriate site when symptoms fail to respond as expected

A well-planned and coordinated approach to emergency and hospital treatment will achieve the best success in helping your child get back to good health.

10

Asthma and Your Family

Six-year-old Sasha was recently diagnosed with asthma in the emergency room where she was treated and sent home with a prescription. At a follow-up visit to the pediatrician, Sasha's parents asked what else they could do—in addition to giving her medicine—to help to prevent future asthma attacks.

To offer specific advice, the doctor needed to learn something about Sasha's home environment. Her parents explained that they live in an apartment that has wall-to-wall carpeting throughout. The carpet is vacuumed weekly, but it is quite old. Sasha's bedroom has bunk beds and shelves full of stuffed animals. The windows have both miniblinds and drapes. From this description, the physician was able to make suggestions for removing potential asthma triggers from Sasha's home.

This chapter offers recommendations for eliminating common triggers so that you can do the same for your child at home. And it discusses typical family issues, such as behavior, communication, and relationships with your child who has asthma as well as with siblings, relatives, and caregivers.

ASTHMA-PROOFING YOUR HOME

As you work to achieve better control of your child's asthma, it is important to asthma-proof your home by eliminating triggers that can lead to flares. If your child has been skin-tested for allergies, you can make specific changes in his bedroom and the rest of the house to minimize contact with the offending allergen. Even if your child hasn't been tested for allergies, these suggestions can help all children with asthma reduce or eliminate possible triggers that can cause airway inflammation.

Most children have year-round symptoms that are commonly affected by indoor asthma triggers, so you can best reduce those triggers if you know what they are and where to find them. Earlier chapters explained that the most common indoor triggers are dust mites, mold, cockroaches, rodents, animal dander, and secondhand tobacco smoke. Other triggers, such as strong smells from perfumes or cleaners, physical exercise, increased humidity, low temperatures, and houseplants or greenery, such as live Christmas trees, also affect some children.

The most important part of your home to target asthma triggers is the place where your child spends much of his time, both awake and asleep. For most children it's the bedroom, but it may also be the living room, family room, or wherever they spend a lot of time playing, watching television, or using a computer. First, here are some recommendations for the whole house, then some specific suggestions for your child's room.

Around the House

Changes that are easy to make and inexpensive can be made throughout the home:

- Keep your home smoke-free.
- Remove carpets where possible. Ideally, it's best to remove carpets throughout the home, but at least take them out of your child's bedroom. Cleaning solutions (e.g., DustMiteX, Allersearch ADS, and

Allersearch X-Mite cleaner) are available for reducing house dust mites, but they don't eliminate the presence of mold spores in carpeting, which can be an asthma trigger.

- Fix leaky faucets. Stagnant water can attract roaches, increase humidity, and lead to mildew and mold.
- Reduce humidity in the house to less than 50 percent by using dehumidifiers or central air conditioners. If you don't have central air, a window air conditioner unit is preferable to a window fan, which can pull pollen into the house. Use a dehumidifier in the basement to reduce mold exposure. Avoid belt-type humidifiers because bacteria and fungi thrive on the damp belts.
- Dust furniture weekly.
- Wipe down baseboards with hot water and soap on a weekly basis to reduce dust mites and remove pieces and feces of cockroaches, which are potent allergens.
- Vacuum when your child is out of the house to avoid dust inhalation.
- Never leave food out. Keep food and garbage in closed containers. Seal garbage and take it out at the end of the day to reduce cockroaches and rodents.
- Place roach and mice bait in childproof containers and out of the reach of your child. If a spray is used to kill roaches, she should stay out of the room until the odor goes away.
- Select vinyl or leather coverings the next time you buy upholstered furniture. It isn't necessary to throw out a cloth-covered stuffed sofa, but you might buy an inexpensive vinyl-covered beanbag chair for your child to sit in while watching TV. That way, she'll be less exposed to dust than if she snuggles into a sofa pillow.
- Install ventilators (exhaust fans) for appliances like stoves when possible.
- Keep your heating system and its filters well maintained.
- Use nonallergenic cleaning products (ammonia, baking soda, beeswax, lemon oil, mineral oil, paste wax, nonchlorine bleaches, white or apple cider vinegar mixed with water).
- Avoid scented and deodorant soaps. Choose mild soaps instead.

In Your Child's Bedroom

Most children spend about fifty to sixty hours a week sleeping and even more time playing or hanging out in their bedrooms. One of the most important steps you can take to remove common asthma triggers is to target your child's bedroom aggressively. This doesn't mean you must scrub everything twice a day; most of these changes are not difficult or time-consuming. For example:

- Cover pillows, mattresses, and box springs in plastic or dust-filtering covers; pillows should be made of washable, synthetic material, not feathers.

- Use washable, synthetic blankets; avoid fuzzy cotton or wool blankets.

- Bedding, including pillows, should be washed once a week in hot water (hotter than 130 degrees) to kill dust mites.

- If you have pets, keep them outdoors if possible. Keep them out of your child's room at all times and keep the bedroom door shut.

- Replace venetian blinds or miniblinds and fabric curtains (that attract and hold dust) with smooth, pull-down shades that are easily wiped down with warm, soapy water. It's even better if you can replace all blinds and drapes with shades throughout your home.

- Replace any carpet (wall-to-wall or area rugs) in your child's room with a bare wood floor or tile that can be damp-mopped regularly.

- Keep clothes in drawers and/or closets with the closet door shut. Keep any woolen clothing in heavy plastic bags.

- Clean or dust surfaces in your child's room weekly. Try to use furniture that doesn't attract and hold dust (wood, metal, or plastic as opposed to upholstered when possible). Avoid shelves that hold pictures, books, and knickknacks; move those items to another room or store them in closed cabinets.

- Contain clutter. Although it's difficult to remove clutter from any child's bedroom, it is essential—every night—to put all toys and books in closed containers, drawers, or closets. This reduces your child's exposure to dust while sleeping.
- Avoid stuffed animals. It's hard for children to give up stuffed creatures completely, but try to keep them to a minimum. At least keep them off the bed. If your child has a favorite stuffed animal, wash it regularly in hot water.
- Keep all food out of your child's room to avoid attracting roaches.
- If your home has a forced-air heating system, turn it off in your child's room, or cover the bedroom air vents with filters.

Many places sell supplies that help reduce allergens in the bedroom. Most linen or bedding stores carry hypoallergenic mattress and pillow covers. They can also be purchased from online or catalog stores. Some useful items include: electrostatic cloths that remove most dust, HEPA filters to remove animal dander in the air, and a dust mite reducing solution.

THE PET QUESTION

Children with asthma are often allergic to pets that shed hair, dander, and feathers. Some studies indicate that if pets are present in the home before the diagnosis of asthma, a child may already be sensitized to pets and less likely to be allergic to them. Once a child has been diagnosed with asthma, however, it is better to avoid furry and feathered pets. If you don't remove a pet from your home, at least keep it out of your child's bedroom *at all times*, even when your child isn't in his room. Animal dander is very sticky, so if a furry pet lives in your home, every effort should be made to wipe down all surfaces each week.

While this can be very difficult, it is important to keep your child from picking up and playing with the animal. Acceptable options for pets include fish, reptiles, frogs, or turtles.

SMOKE

Tobacco smoke is the most common irritant for children with asthma. The best way to reduce tobacco smoke pollution exposure in the home is for the smoker to stop smoking. If there is a smoker in your family who has not completely quit smoking, the next best goal is to move the smoke away from your child who has asthma.

Steps to a Smoke-Free Home

Children with asthma are at a higher risk from the effects of cigarette smoke. Parents can take these steps to protect their children:

- Smoke only in one room
- Blow smoke out the window
- Use an air purifier or smoke filter
- Never smoke near a child
- Never smoke in a car with a child
- Smoke only outside the home
- Never allow smoke in your home or car
- Never allow smoke around a child
- Quit smoking

Even if no one smokes in your home, don't forget to speak to your child's caretakers (baby-sitters, relatives, friends' parents, neighbors, a parent who carpools and smokes in the car) about the importance of avoiding environmental tobacco smoke. Identify other places where your child may be exposed to tobacco smoke. If your child is old enough to understand, talk with him about appropriate steps he can take himself to avoid smoke exposure.

If parents or caretakers continue to smoke, they should always smoke outside and wear a "smoking jacket" that they keep away from the child when they come back into the house. Many adults assume that if they "just step outside" to smoke that they're protecting a child from smoke exposure. But smoke residue settles on their clothing, skin, and hair, and they bring it back inside. If they smoke several times a day, these adults are actually contributing a considerable amount of smoke allergen to a child's environment. Smoke from a fireplace or wood-burning stove may also cause a child to wheeze.

COMMUNICATION

Good communication within the family is essential to manage asthma successfully. Open, honest communication may prevent resentment among family members as well as prevent catastrophic events. For example, sometimes relatives don't take a child's asthma seriously enough, even when they are solely responsible for his care. They may forget to give a child his medicine or pay little attention to his asthma symptoms. They may not think that the medicine is helping, or they are concerned that the child will become dependent on it or habituated to it.

Communicating important information to responsible family members is a valuable starting point. They should understand that asthma is a chronic disease. They should appreciate the importance of avoiding common and specific asthma triggers. And they must know how to treat acute attacks.

Your child's written asthma management plan should be easily accessible and understandable to all family members and other caretakers whenever they are responsible for looking after your child.

Basic information that every responsible relative and caregiver should know includes:

- What daily controller medicines your child uses—the name of the medicine, the dose, and when, how, and why he takes it
- What quick-relief medicines your child uses—the name of the medicine, the dose, and when, how, and why to use it
- Where these medicines are located in your home
- The symptoms of an asthma flare
- What to do to treat a flare
- When and how to get emergency help

Feelings and Family Members

Other members of the family are often affected by your child's asthma. A family may not be able to keep a pet, for example, which affects all members of the family. Holding family meetings to talk about feelings or having one-to-one conversations between parents and siblings of the child with asthma can be very helpful. You can address sibling resentment by making the management of your child's asthma a team effort with everyone doing his or her part to keep your child healthy. All members of the family should attend asthma education classes or occasionally accompany your child to a medical visit to learn more about asthma. Even when there's little or no resentment about the limits asthma may put on your family, this team approach could be applied to help the entire family achieve a valuable goal.

Brothers and sisters may have trouble understanding why their sibling with asthma gets all the attention. When two children share a room, for instance, problems can arise. The child without asthma may not be very happy about having to keep his toys in another room or jammed into the closet each night. He may want to sleep on the top bunk, even though his brother with asthma should sleep up there to avoid having tiny particles of dust rain down on the lower bunk.

"Why do I have to clean my room and you never make her? She always gets out of vacuuming her room!" is a common sibling complaint. A child with asthma has to stay away from things like dust, so her siblings may feel she's being pampered by getting out of household chores.

When the whole family has to cancel an activity because the child with asthma is having a flare, the other children will naturally be angry and resentful. This is a difficult problem for every parent. Your child with asthma probably is getting more of your time and attention than your other children because she's not feeling well. Explain the situation to brothers and sisters as matter-of-factly and honestly as you can. This will help them realize why they all need to help keep asthma triggers down. And it will also help them understand that the sibling with asthma isn't deliberately having flares just to ruin everyone's day. Look for compromise solutions that fairly satisfy everyone as much as possible.

A child with asthma might not be able to help with the vacuuming or dusting, for example, but there are always dishes to wash.

Communication with a Child Who Has Asthma

As your child grows older, she may start to resent not being "normal." She doesn't like missing school or being away from her friends because she has a doctor's appointment or is having a flare. And she probably doesn't like being reminded to take her medicines.

Allow your child to communicate her frustrations. Help her work through these feelings by using problem-solving activities that will encourage her to continue controlling her asthma. For cxample, ask her what happens if she stops taking her everyday medicines? Walk her through the consequences from a mild flare through hospitalization. Then ask her how it feels to be symptom-free when she controls her asthma by taking her medicines.

Most children with asthma feel there is something "different" about them. It is important to discuss these feelings with your child. Allow her to talk about feelings of inadequacy, embarrassment, and other emotions without telling her that she "shouldn't feel that way." Instead of trying to talk her out of her valid emotions, acknowledge her feelings and show that you understand by responding along these lines: "I know you hate to miss basketball practice because you love to play . . ." or "Yes, it's tough when other kids treat you differently . . . ."

Then move on to help him figure out ways that can help him feel less different. Problem-solve with your child ways for dealing with specific situations. For example, some children are self-conscious about using an asthma device at school. Carrying a spacer around can be noticeable by classmates, but a Diskus that fits into a pocket or purse may be more acceptable. Your child can easily use it in a bathroom stall without being noticed.

You could also emphasize that good asthma control will allow your child to do whatever she wants to do without needing to take out the dreaded rescue/quick-relief medicine in public. Help your child set one realistic goal at a time when discussing her asthma management. Talk about what she can do and what you will do to help her reach this goal.

Age-Appropriate Behaviors

Just as children reach milestones in physical growth and development at various ages, their acceptance of asthma as a daily reality in their lives will change with each developmental stage. It is important for parents to understand what reactions to expect. Chapter 12 discusses toddlers, who often resist asthma treatment and are too young to understand its importance. Chapter 13 addresses issues that often arise with teenagers, who naturally want to become more independent and may decide they don't need medicines any longer.

Whatever your child's age, keep in mind that her reactions and behaviors will change as she grows and develops. Your expectations about her responses to having asthma will need to be flexible enough to adapt to her feelings and behaviors. But one constant remains: as her parent, you will always need to support and encourage her in managing this disease.

ASTHMA AND STRESS

Strong emotional reactions—both positive and negative—may trigger asthma symptoms in some children. Parents often ask whether there's a link between asthma and emotions, particularly those emotions that upset or stress children. Many studies have looked at a possible connection between asthma and stress, but none are conclusive. It appears that there is some link, but the exact nature of such a link is uncertain. Researchers do agree, however, that it is not a simple case of cause and effect. That is, stress doesn't cause asthma, but in some children it may make asthma more difficult to control.

Parents and professionals have observed that shouting from anger or excitement can bring on symptoms in some children with asthma, as can hard crying or a tantrum. Laughing hard can even be a trigger for some youngsters. Strong emotions seem to make some children hyperventi-late: they breathe in and out faster and less deeply. Hyperventilation can make their airways cool off and get dried out, which in turn may trigger an asthma flare.

You can't prevent every situation that could lead to crying or yelling, but try to do whatever you can to keep negative emotions and arguments from escalating into screaming matches. If asthma symptoms are trig-gered by emotionally charged situations, use the quick-relief medicine promptly. You certainly want your child to have fun and laugh. A little tickling is fun, but don't overdo it. Stop before your child starts to get short of breath or cough.

ASTHMA AND SLEEPING

Children with poorly controlled asthma often have symptoms at night. As mentioned previously, it is important to create a trigger-free envi-ronment in your child's bedroom. You can go a step further: *where* your child sleeps in the bedroom can also affect asthma triggers. In Sasha's case, for example, when her family discovered that cold air triggers her asthma, they moved her bed away from the window. She loves her bunk beds, but her parents make sure that she always sleeps on the top bunk; if she slept on the lower bunk, she would have greater exposure to dust mites from the mattress above.

If nighttime coughing makes your child wake up more than twice a month, let your doctor or nurse practitioner know. This usually means that she needs to be on another medicine or a higher dose of the medi-cine that she is currently taking.

Make sure that the quick-relief medicine is easily accessible by you or your child, depending on her age. Sleepless nights usually lead to less productive days, especially in school-aged children. If coughing has made your child lose sleep, make sure she is physically well enough to go to school the next day. If she is, let the teacher or school nurse know that she had some coughing during the night and may be a little sleepy the following day. You do not need to keep your child home unless she is having symptoms in the morning.

Remember that a child whose asthma is well controlled should not need more than two canisters of quick-relief medicine (albuterol) in a year. If your child requires more than this because of nighttime symptoms, contact your child's doctor right away.

FAMILY LIFE

Every child's participation in family life includes helping out with chores. There's no reason children with asthma should be excused from these responsibilities. They should be able to participate in:

- Washing dishes
- Damp-mopping floors
- Baby-sitting
- Cooking
- Setting and clearing the table
- Drying dishes and putting them away
- Sorting and folding laundry
- Food shopping and putting groceries away
- Washing the family car
- Sewing or mending

But certain chores may trigger asthma flares and should be avoided. These include:

- Vacuuming
- Frying foods
- Dusting
- Cleaning with strong-smelling cleaners
- Brushing or washing pets
- Mowing grass
- Raking leaves

Children with asthma can participate in many physical activities that families do together. Encourage activities that your family will enjoy.

Most children can play any sport if they take the right medicine and keep their asthma under control. Many Olympic athletes have asthma (see the list in Resources) and are able to excel in their chosen sport because their asthma is controlled. Be aware, however, that a child with asthma will need to warm up slowly for high-level activities. When you participate in family sport activities together, do warm-up exercises with your child.

Other nonphysical family activities that may be equally enjoyable include going to movies, museums, and amusement parks in tobacco smoke–free environments. In general, your child should avoid hayrides, zoos, and park outings in high pollen seasons.

Vacations should be planned with the entire family's input, but it is important to choose an environment that will be less likely to trigger an asthma episode. Clearly if your child gets sick on the vacation, no one is going to have much fun.

ASTHMA AND BEHAVIOR

Sometimes a child may try to take advantage of his asthma to get extra days off from school or avoid chores and other responsibilities. At school, he may try to get out of gym class or other activities he doesn't like.

You don't want to reward a child for these behaviors when they're not genuine. At the same time, you want to be sure you are taking his asthma seriously. It's not always easy to tell whether his complaints are real or an excuse, but here's a general guideline: be firm and consistent, and don't reward him for being sick. If he's home with an asthma flare, for example, give him the attention he needs, but don't turn a sick day into a fun day by treating him to extra presents or food treats that send the message that being sick is a pleasant event.

Some youngsters think of asthma as a serious handicap that makes them sick all the time. They may feel they're different from their classmates or "not as good." They may have trouble making friends, especially if they have to miss a lot of school or can't participate in after-school sports and other activities. They may be more concerned about what they can't do because of their asthma than what they *can* do.

Once your child's asthma is under control, most of the reasons for his negative feelings will disappear. He'll still be a little different because he has asthma, but in most other ways he'll be just like every other child. As his health improves, help him focus on what he can do and encourage him to become gradually more active.

WHEN TO KEEP YOUR CHILD AT HOME

Parents often find it difficult to decide whether to keep a child home from day care or school, in part because it usually means Mom or Dad will lose a day of work. If you've spotted symptoms early and have immediately started taking the treatment steps in your child's asthma management plan, it's probably okay to send him to school. Just be sure he will get his medicine on schedule at day care or school.

In general, your child should *not* go to school when any of the following situations apply:

- When he had a restless night due to coughing or wheezing
- When he is having difficulty breathing and is not responding to quick-relief medicines
- When he is using neck, stomach, and rib muscles to breathe
- When you are uncomfortable about how he is breathing

You should consider keeping your child home:

- When he needs quick-relief medicines more than every six hours
- When there is a field trip that will expose him to known asthma triggers (unless you can make other arrangements)

It is usually *not* necessary to keep your child home:

- When he has a scratchy throat

- When he is in the early stages of a cold
- When he shows early allergy season signs

If you're in doubt, it is probably best to keep him home for the first few hours and call your doctor's office. For an older child who has established his personal best, you may use the peak flow meter reading to help determine whether he should stay home. If the reading is getting lower, or if it is in the red or danger zone, he should be taken to see a doctor immediately. Unfortunately the peak flow meter is effort-dependent, which means that if your child doesn't want to do well on the peak flow meter, he won't.

The opposite situation may also arise. That is, your child says he feels fine but you can see symptoms. He might do all he can to avoid school, but when it comes to playing or an activity he really wants to do, he may insist he's perfectly okay—even when he's wheezing. For an older child, the peak flow meter may help you determine if he is having trouble breathing. If his reading is normal, he can play outdoors; if it's below normal, it's time for quiet, indoor activities. With younger children, watch them breathe while they're engaged in some activity. If you notice that they're working harder to breathe while they play, you may want to direct them to quieter activities.

Some parents use pollen counts as a measurement guide for staying indoors when the child has demonstrated pollen sensitivity (itchy nose; watery, runny eyes; sneezing). Decide with your child on a cutoff point, and you should both agree on what you will accept as a reliable source for pollen count information. Below the cutoff, he can play outdoors; above it, it's better to play indoors.

Cutoff numbers can be useful guides, but they vary with individuals—there isn't a definite number for all children—so parents have to rely on common sense and their child's past experience with pollen-related symptoms when using pollen counts to determine outdoor or indoor limits. Unfortunately, the pollen counts reported by TV, radio, the Web, and newspapers usually lag behind today's pollen by a day or two. A good Web site for interpretation of accurate pollen counts approved by the American Academy of Allergy, Asthma and Immunology is www.aaaai.org/nab/index.cfm?p=reading_charts.

ASTHMA MANAGEMENT PLAN: MAKING IT WORK AT HOME

A key lesson of this book cannot be emphasized enough: an asthma management plan is essential to help you monitor your child's use of medicines. It is important to place the written plan where both you and your child can see it. When your child feels that it's time to begin the asthma management plan for a flare, he should let you know. Whenever you have a new baby-sitter or caretaker in your home, be sure to point out the plan, review it to be sure it's understood correctly, and point out where medicines are located. It is also important to take your child's plan with you to every medical visit and review it with your physician or nurse practitioner.

With these suggestions, your home can be a healthier, more trigger-free environment, and your entire family will be more confident about controlling your child's asthma.

11

Asthma, Sports, and Exercise

One of the more common asthma myths is that someone with asthma cannot or should not exercise or participate in sports. Nothing could be further from the truth. Exercise is—or should be—a part of daily life. Children, teenagers, and adults with asthma should be able to enjoy any aspect of life they choose, including hiking, biking, basketball, ballet, soccer, gymnastics, and other physical activities.

Many Olympic athletes who have asthma have won gold medals in a wide variety of sports, from swimming to figure skating to track and field (see Resources). Every professional sport has at least one present or future hall of fame athlete who has asthma. Across the country, millions of people with asthma, from the five-year-old soccer player to the eighty-five-year-old marathon runner, take part in sports without being limited by their disease. They can enjoy, participate, and compete in physical activities as long as they have their asthma under control.

EXERCISE-INDUCED ASTHMA

The most common form of asthma is *exercise-induced* asthma— a slightly misleading term because exercise *doesn't cause* asthma.

Exercise can bring out symptoms because of the increased demands placed on a person's breathing while running, jumping, swimming, skating, skiing, or other forms of physical exertion.

When our bodies are at rest, we inhale and exhale a certain number of times at a certain volume. As we breathe through our nose (the body's "air treatment intake valve"), the air is warmed and humidified before it gets to the lungs. When we exercise, our muscles need more oxygen and produce more carbon dioxide than they do when we're resting or inactive. Since we take in oxygen and get rid of carbon dioxide by breathing, we have to increase our air exchange by breathing deeper and faster while we exercise. We also breathe through our mouths instead of our noses so we can move as much air as possible into and out of our lungs. When we breathe this way during exercise, the air in our lungs is cooler and drier than usual.

Researchers who study exercise-induced asthma believe that this cooler, drier air stimulates inflammatory cells in our airways. Once stimulated, these cells release chemicals called *mediators*. Some mediators make the airways swell or produce mucus, while other mediators irritate the muscles that encircle the airways and make them tighten up. As a result, the airways become narrow or constricted. The narrowed airways limit the amount of air that can come in or go out—right at the time when the body needs more air, not less. When oxygen delivery decreases and carbon dioxide levels increase, the muscles tire more quickly, and the athlete with uncontrolled asthma has to stop physical exertion.

In most cases, asthma symptoms brought on by exercise occur about five minutes after the exertion begins. Chest tightness is a common first symptom, along with shortness of breath. The athlete is usually forced to slow down or stop, and may bend forward at the waist to help force air out of the lungs. Wheezing and coughing usually follow. The symptoms decrease with rest, but they may come back when exercise is resumed.

SYMPTOM PREVENTION

The key to exercise or sports participation for anyone with asthma is to prevent the process that leads to airway narrowing. Traditionally, a bronchodilator is prescribed for use before exertion. This medicine is usually given by a metered dose inhaler (MDI) and a spacer. The bronchodilator works by relaxing muscles that surround the airways. When they are relaxed, the muscles can't squeeze the airways, and the airways stay open.

Although this seems to work to some degree for many people, a bronchodilator before exercise may not be the most complete treatment because a bronchodilator does not treat inflammation. The swelling and mucus in the airways, therefore, can still be a problem. The bronchodilator-before-exercise treatment plan also does not cover the possibility of spontaneous exercise that is common among children, such as running outside to play ball with friends or racing to catch the school bus.

It is likely that many people who only have asthma symptoms with exercise have a low level of inflammation in their airways. In other words, their inflammation is not enough to cause symptoms while their bodies are at rest, but they do come on with exercise. These individuals may also experience mild symptoms during other times of biological stress, such as when they catch a cold. If this low-level inflammation exists, there may be long-term consequences as well. Some asthma researchers believe that constant inflammation can cause permanent damage to the airways. No studies have yet been done, however, to find out if there is long-term lung damage in people with asthma whose symptoms are brought on *only* with physical exertion.

The possibility of low-level airway inflammation raises this question: Should people whose symptoms only occur with exercise take a daily anti-inflammatory medicine? This therapy would decrease or eliminate the inflammation. Daily anti-inflammatory therapy would also allow for better tolerance of spontaneous exertion. It might also increase their breathing capacity more than if they used only a bronchodilator before exercising. Consider Scott's situation:

> Whenever ten-year-old Scott exercised, he coughed, wheezed, and had chest tightness and shortness of breath. He had occasional wheezing in the spring, but otherwise he had no symptoms or complaints. He used a bronchodilator when springtime symptoms appeared. As a competitive swimmer, he also used it before swim practice and team meets.

Halfway through the swimming season, his doctor suggested that Scott try an anti-inflammatory medicine, even though he had no symptoms. After a few weeks, his coaches noticed that Scott was swimming several seconds faster. Scott also became aware that he was able to swim faster for longer distances. His parents, however, did not renew the prescription for the anti-inflammatory medicine because Scott seemed better. Two weeks after stopping the medicine, Scott's times fell back to where they were before he started the medicine. Scott also noticed the change and asked his parents if he could restart the anti-inflammatory medicine. Within two weeks of restarting the daily therapy, Scott was again swimming faster.

While daily anti-inflammatory therapy might improve the athlete's performance, there is the increased cost of daily therapy in both time and money. Different health care professionals treat asthma differently, and each individual with asthma is unique. If your child has asthma symptoms when exercising or playing sports, talk to your doctor or nurse practitioner about whether a daily anti-inflammatory treatment is right for your child.

BEFORE EXERCISING

If a bronchodilator is prescribed for use before exercise, it must be taken at least fifteen minutes before the exercise begins to be as effective as possible. A long, slow warm-up, such as easy running or swimming, before the actual practice, game, or event begins, may also decrease symptoms during exercise. In cold weather, wearing a scarf or trying to breathe through the nose during the early part of the exercise may help as well. Quick-relief medicines along with any necessary delivery equipment should be available during and after the exercise in case symptoms do arise.

Young athletes with asthma may still seem to have symptoms even though therapy is being used. If symptoms occur when they are using only a bronchodilator before exercise, then it may be a sign that airway inflammation is present. Adding a daily anti-inflammatory medicine may decrease symptoms. If they are already using anti-inflammatory therapy and symptoms continue during exercise, a stronger medicine may be needed. Sometimes if a child with asthma has a cold, is having problems with allergies, or is having a mild asthma flare, then the airways will be more sensitive and symptoms during exercise will occur more readily. Limiting exercise on these days may be necessary.

WHAT OTHER ADULTS SHOULD KNOW

Coaches and gym teachers should be aware that your child has asthma and should allow him or her to stop, rest, or take quick-relief medicines if symptoms occur. Hopefully, this can be done without bringing too much attention to a child with asthma because it can affect self-esteem or cause embarrassment. Coaches and school nurses should know how to administer the medicines if necessary. Give a copy of your child's asthma management plan to coaches and teachers and review it with them.

CONDITIONING

Despite adequate therapy, shortness of breath with exercise may continue. This symptom could indicate a lower level of fitness, which can be remedied by physical conditioning. Children and teenagers who were less active when their asthma was not well controlled have usually limited their exercise in general. Their muscles are therefore not used to the sustained demands of, for example, a competitive game of soccer, fast-break basketball, or a long, uphill hike.

Some children and adults with asthma develop a sedentary lifestyle from an early age and may be overweight. But gradual physical conditioning—that builds increased strength and endurance—can have life-long benefits not just for their lungs but also for their entire bodies. Young athletes will sometimes need to be patient and condition their bodies by gradually increasing their degree of activity until they can participate to their full potential.

ASTHMA AND WEIGHT

Some researchers have noted a relationship between asthma and a tendency to be overweight or obese, but the connection is not clear. It may be that children with asthma are not as physically active, either because their asthma is not under good control or because their parents limit their activity. It may be possible, however, that obesity is a risk factor for developing asthma. In either case, overweight or obese children and adolescents with asthma seem to have more problems not only with their asthma but also with other diseases.

Successful treatment of an overweight child or adolescent involves both moderate exercise and a nutritious diet. Running, bicycling, swimming, or even vigorous walking for twenty minutes three times a week—along with a diet that minimizes junk food—can result in gradual, safe weight loss. Obesity is a medical condition itself and is best treated by a weight management program that is supervised by medical professionals.

Not every child is destined to be an athlete, but exercise is an important part of health maintenance for all young people. Children should be able to play and participate in sports without worrying about breathing. Controlling asthma will help your child enjoy an active, healthy lifestyle.

12

Infants and Toddlers with Asthma

The wheezing infant has confused health professionals for years. Many physician training programs taught that a child should not be diagnosed as having asthma before the age of two or, in some instances, age four. Other terms such as "reactive airways disease," "chronic bronchitis," or "recurrent bronchiolitis" were used to describe infants and toddlers with recurring cough, wheezing, or labored breathing.

The current definition of asthma does not exclude any age group. In fact, guidelines from the National Institutes of Health make specific mention of the infant and toddler with asthma. The diagnosis of asthma is based not on age but on a child's medical history and physical examination. If an infant or toddler meets the criteria and other possible diseases are excluded, the child is diagnosed with asthma. Yet there are some differences between infants and toddlers with asthma and older children and adults with asthma. Parents need to understand the special considerations for this youngest age group.

THE COLD CONNECTION

Many different types of triggers can cause an asthma flare in older children and adults. In infants and toddlers, however, the most common trigger is a cold caused by a respiratory virus, known as a "viral upper respiratory tract infection," or URI. The usual pattern for an infant with asthma starts with a cold, then the cough gets worse, and finally labored breathing and wheezing begin. In young children whose asthma is not well controlled, other nonspecific irritants such as smoke or fumes can also trigger asthma symptoms. Allergies play a smaller role in these early years, although some children show allergic tendencies quite early in life.

Studies of the development of asthma have followed a large group of children from birth. These studies suggest that babies and toddlers with asthma fall into two categories:

GROUP ONE

The first group has asthma symptoms until age four or so and then no longer shows any symptoms. These infants and toddlers have asthma symptoms only with colds and have none when they are well. Parents of children in this group tend *not* to have asthma. Children in this group usually don't have any signs of allergies, such as eczema. This is the only group that seems to "outgrow" asthma. Young children who have asthma symptoms only with colds might be treated with asthma medicines from the first sign of a cold until the last symptom is gone, and they may not need to take controller medicines in between. Consider this child's situation:

> Brenda got her first cold when she was two months old. The first day she had a runny nose, then she started coughing. The next day the runny nose disappeared, but the cough grew worse in severity and occurred during sleep. She also developed a "rattle" in her chest. Her cough continued for two weeks despite cough medicine and then gradually went away. She caught another cold a month

later and almost immediately developed a hacking cough and chest congestion. Her pediatrician heard wheezing and prescribed albuterol by nebulizer. The albuterol helped temporarily, but her symptoms returned four hours later. These symptoms hung on for two weeks before disappearing. This pattern continued through a few more colds.

During a well-baby visit, Brenda's pediatrician prescribed an inhaled steroid to go along with the albuterol and advised her parents to start the medicines at the first sign of a cold. A month later, they began giving her medicines the first day her nose started running. This time her cough only lasted three days and seemed less severe. This plan was used for each cold, and the cough and wheezing were easily controlled.

In the spring following Brenda's third birthday, her doctor recommended stopping this plan. Brenda had several minor colds over the next few years, but the harsh cough and wheezing never returned.

In youngsters like Brenda, asthma symptoms appear only with colds. Using a quick-relief medicine alone (albuterol) decreases the symptoms for the moment, but they return over two weeks. Adding an anti-inflammatory medicine (the inhaled steroid) to the albuterol at the first sign of a cold controls symptoms so they are not as severe and do not last long. This plan may work in some cases, but in other cases a child may need to take an anti-inflammatory medicine every day—even when well—to prevent asthma symptoms during colds.

GROUP TWO

In the second category, infants and toddlers have symptoms not only during colds but also in between colds. Parents of children in this group usually have a history of asthma, and these children are more likely to show some form of allergic disease. They do not outgrow their asthma, although there may be periods of remission later in life. Some children in this group also experience a decline in lung function.

Young children who have symptoms in between colds benefit from daily controller therapy to guard against the inflammation that causes symptoms. Children in this group tend to have symptoms that are more severe and more difficult to control. Daily controller medicines may also guard against loss of lung function. Compare Brenda's case with Michael's below:

> Four-month-old Michael developed a hacking cough, wheezing, and labored breathing after getting his first cold. His mother, who has had asthma all of her life, recognized the symptoms immediately and took her son to the doctor's office. Michael was admitted to the hospital with "bronchiolitis" and treated with nebulized albuterol and oral prednisone. He was discharged with a nebulizer, and his parents were given instructions to give albuterol by nebulizer if the wheezing returned.
>
> In the months following the hospitalization, Michael had several wheezing episodes. The albuterol made the wheezing disappear for a time. He also developed eczema. With the next cold, Michael had severe labored breathing despite several albuterol treatments and was hospitalized again. This time, he was diagnosed with asthma, and a daily inhaled steroid was prescribed as maintenance therapy. Two weeks later, the episodic wheezing stopped.
>
> With each cold, he experienced three to five days of harsh coughing and wheezing, but these symptoms were easily relieved with albuterol. Throughout his school-age and teen years, Michael continued to have brief, mild bouts of wheezing in response to a variety of triggers, and his symptoms got worse whenever the daily medicines were withdrawn.

His mother's history of asthma, the appearance of eczema, and his wheezing in between colds suggested that Michael would have persistent asthma beyond infancy. Children like Michael need daily anti-inflammatory therapy to decrease symptoms, prevent asthma flares, and maintain good lung function.

When your infant or toddler is diagnosed as having asthma, keep in mind that he has about a fifty-fifty chance of "outgrowing" asthma. The chances of outgrowing it are better if all of the following are true:

- Your child only wheezes with colds.
- Neither parent has asthma (diagnosed by a physician).
- Your child does not have eczema (diagnosed by a physician).
- Your child does not have other signs of allergies.

No matter which group your child is in, he may need daily controller therapy with an anti-inflammatory medicine. You must also have an asthma management plan to use when your child has symptoms, even if daily medicine is not prescribed. You should be able to evaluate your young child for wheezing or labored breathing, because infants and toddlers cannot tell you how they feel or describe their symptoms.

Remember: a wheeze is a continuous musical noise when a child breathes out. Signs of labored breathing include breathing fast, flaring nostrils, and when the skin in between the ribs and underneath the rib cage seems to get sucked in, a sign called *retractions*. Review these signs with your child's doctor or nurse practitioner so you can recognize them early and act promptly.

USING THE NEBULIZER WITH INFANTS AND TODDLERS

Infants are usually treated with inhaled medicines given by nebulizer at first. Parents generally learn how to use nebulizers easily, and young infants quickly accept them. It takes several minutes, however, to deliver medicine with nebulizers. Older infants and toddlers may not want to sit still for that period of time. Nebulizers can also be inefficient in terms of medicine delivery. In order to get the most benefit from the medicine, young children should wear a face mask while receiving the treatment, rather than using the "blow-by" method.

Metered dose inhalers (MDIs) can be used to deliver inhaled medicines to infants and toddlers by using a valved holding chamber with a mask. Although this method requires more training for parents, it takes less time and delivers the medicine more efficiently than a nebulizer.

With either method, it may take some time for a child to become comfortable with the mask, especially a child between one and two years of age. When an infant or toddler fights the mask, it might be due to a fear of the mask, a poor mask fit, or applying the treatment at an inopportune time, such as when she's fussy or wants to be more active.

You can help your infant or toddler get used to the mask by letting her play with it and by gentle, brief applications during nontreatment times. The mask should fit easily over her mouth and nose but should not extend above the bridge of her nose or below her chin. It might take several days of persistent mask application before a young child starts to accept the treatment with any consistency.

Choosing the treatment time is important. The treatment can be given more effectively while a child is sleeping or during "quiet times" when you are reading to her or watching television than at times when she's cranky or unwilling to sit still.

DO SYMPTOMS ALWAYS MEAN ASTHMA?

The airways of infants are small, and other conditions besides asthma can cause wheezing. In young infants, an infection from a virus can cause coughs, wheezing, or labored breathing. The *respiratory syncytial virus*, or RSV, is the most common virus that can cause these symptoms in young infants, although other viruses can do the same thing. RSV usually appears in the late fall or winter. Some researchers believe that RSV infection can cause a child to develop asthma, while others think that RSV triggers asthma that was already present.

Since viral infections are the most common trigger of asthma flares in infants and toddlers, it is difficult to tell whether a first episode of wheezing is from the infection or from asthma. When wheezing or other symptoms keep coming back with every cold, however, it is more likely because the child has asthma.

Other disorders can cause asthma symptoms in young children. Gastroesophageal reflux, also called acid reflux, can lead to coughing and wheezing in some babies. This condition causes acid from the stomach to travel back up the esophagus, the tube that connects the mouth to the stomach. The esophagus is sensitive, and the acid sometimes irritates nerve endings in the esophagus and triggers coughing or wheezing. Sometimes stomach contents travel all the way up to the back of the throat and irritate the airway, again causing coughing or wheezing.

Acid reflux is easy to detect in young infants who spit up or have wet burps. But in older infants and toddlers, testing may be needed to detect it. The presence of acid reflux in infants or toddlers with asthma makes it more difficult to control their asthma.

Cystic fibrosis is another disorder that produces some of the same symptoms as asthma. Cystic fibrosis is a genetic disease that is most common in Caucasians. Your doctor may request testing to rule out this disease.

When asthma is not properly diagnosed or treated in a very young child, the quality of life for the whole family suffers. A prompt diagnosis and an appropriate treatment plan, however, will leave everyone in the family free to embrace the ordinary trials, tribulations, and joys of infancy and toddlerhood.

13

Teenagers with Asthma

Darren's asthma was diagnosed when he was seven. Until he was twelve or thirteen, his asthma was well controlled. He followed a daily routine of taking his controller medicine twice a day. It became a mechanical event, like dressing in the morning and undressing at night. He and his family knew certain triggers to avoid, and they kept his room fairly clean and dust free. Darren rarely had a flare.

But by ninth grade, he began to wheeze frequently, especially at night. His parents noticed that he was using his quick-relief inhaler more often. When Darren was due for a routine physical exam, they urged him to tell his doctor about the change in his symptoms.

Darren's body was growing, but his increasing symptoms had more to do with becoming an adolescent than as a result of any physical changes. He was "just being a teenager," and that behavior altered how he managed his asthma. Darren became

*careless about taking his controller medicine as he stuffed
homework in his backpack and dashed for the school bus in the
mornings. At night, he often fell asleep in his clothes before
remembering to take his medicine. He was out and about with
friends more often, hiking through the woods, trying a cigarette
once in a while, visiting homes of classmates who had dogs and
cats, hanging out in their damp basement rec rooms, . . . all
typical preteen activities, but in settings where asthma triggers
thrived.*

WHAT'S "NORMAL" ADOLESCENCE?

As any child with a chronic condition enters adolescence, parents need
to look at the broad picture—what it means to be a typical teenager. An
adolescent with asthma goes through the same emotional, social, and
developmental changes that occur with all teenagers. Those changes
will influence the way he deals with his disease. So let's look at the
background first.

Adolescence is the period of transition between childhood and adulthood, but it isn't bracketed by rigid starting and ending dates. No child
suddenly becomes a teenager on his thirteenth birthday or graduates
from adolescence on his eighteenth. Adolescence can start anytime after
age ten, and some young people become responsible and independent
earlier than eighteen, the legal age of adulthood. Others continue to have
adolescent behaviors into their twenties or thirties. Adolescents are at an
age when they become more aware of themselves as individuals, try to
figure out where they fit in society, and continue to gain the skills they
need to become adults. They want to become more independent from
parents. They are concerned about peer acceptance as they grow away
from their immediate families and develop a second "family" of friends
and classmates. During this period, teenagers develop a new interest in
their bodies as well.

A major characteristic of adolescents is their focus on short-term outcomes; long-term goals and consequences are fuzzy. They think in concrete, immediate terms and are not yet completely able to think abstractly. For this reason, teenagers usually don't worry about long-term health issues. For example, if you tell teens that smoking is bad for their health because it increases their risk of heart disease and cancer in thirty to forty years, you'll get a blank stare. But tell them that smoking stains their teeth, makes their hair and clothes reek, and makes their breath smell bad, and they are more likely to listen because these consequences are immediate and concrete.

If a teenager like Darren is having asthma symptoms, he'll reach for a quick-relief inhaler because he lives in the here and now—he wants immediate relief. That's concrete thinking. But because he's not thinking abstractly about longer-term consequences, he doesn't appreciate the importance of taking controller medicines when he feels well. The result is that he becomes sloppy about taking it regularly.

Adolescents usually want more independence, although they're selective about what they want to be responsible for. Most teenagers want to choose their own clothes, for instance, but may not want the responsibility of paying for them. It's hardly front-page news to say that adolescents tend to rebel against "nonpeer" authority—such as adults who admonish them to be more responsible about taking their medicine.

As physical changes occur in adolescence, parents also need to keep in mind that changing hormone levels often trigger new behaviors. Teenagers are more prone to risk-taking behaviors and are sensitive to peer pressure as well. Just keep in mind that these are all normal developmental stages as you nudge your adolescent toward greater independence and responsibility.

ASTHMA FROM THE TEEN'S POINT OF VIEW

Many characteristics of adolescence can work against a teenager with a chronic disease like asthma. For example, he may fear that having asthma will make him less acceptable to his friends and peers. The need to take daily medicine often makes a teenager feel "different" at a time when it is critically important to fit in and be like other adolescents. (If you don't believe how teenagers desperately want to be like their peers, just walk through a mall and notice how they dress, walk, and talk alike.)

This attitude can lead a teenager to deny that he has asthma or deny the need for daily medicine. Even if he knows and accepts the need for medicine, he may be unwilling to accept the responsibility to take it independently. Although parents, doctors, and nurses recommend that he take controller medicine every day, he may reject the advice simply because it comes from adults. It's not unusual for a teen with asthma to decide he doesn't need medicines any longer. When reminded to take medicine, he may resent parental "interference," ignore it, or not follow through.

At the same time, an adolescent is very aware of the impact of symptoms on his life when asthma flares or is uncontrolled. Coughing can result in unwanted attention—"I hate it when all my classmates turn around and look at me!" Or he may not be able to be as active as he would like. He may get winded quickly on the basketball court and need to sit on the bench, or he may miss school because coughing has kept him awake for several nights and he's exhausted. Teens often become frustrated and depressed when asthma symptoms limit their activities or make them feel different from their peers.

EVERYONE'S GOAL

It is easy for parents and health professionals to become frustrated with a teenager who is bothered by symptoms yet does not take medicines that will control the disease. Adolescents, parents, and health care professionals all need to work together toward the common goal—getting the teenager to manage her disease independently. This means that she becomes responsible for taking daily medicine, recognizing symptoms, and using quick-relief medicines when appropriate. Like adolescence itself, this is a process that may take as long as a few years.

The key to achieving this goal is addressing teens on a common level. Just as adults don't like to follow orders without understanding why they should do so, adolescents are not likely to do something just because an adult "says so." Adults can use teenagers' natural curiosity about their bodies as an opportunity to teach them what asthma is and how they can control their disease. Keep in mind that teens *want* more control over their lives, so capitalize on that desire in motivating them to assume more responsibility for controlling their asthma.

A THREE-STEP PROCESS

Three key steps can help parents guide teenagers toward increasing responsibility. They are *acceptance*, *motivation*, and *action*. These three steps can set the stage for an adolescent to realize that he has a basic choice—he can control his asthma or let it control him.

Acceptance

The first step is to help adolescents accept that they have asthma. Ask your teen what she thinks about having asthma. Help her understand what the disease is, the symptoms it causes, and how it's diagnosed. Health professionals and educational materials can supply the information that a teenager needs in order to accept that she has asthma. You might look for a teen asthma education program in your community. If you don't know of one, ask your asthma care specialist. Teens are often more receptive to learning about asthma from peer groups than from parents or other adults.

Motivation

The next step involves getting your teenager to take more control and responsibility for himself. But how? Lecturing will only fall on deaf ears, so try to engage your teen in a discussion of asthma based on facts, not emotional threats (such as, "If you don't remember your inhaler, you'll end up in the ER again!") or shame ("It's your fault you're wheezing because you didn't take your medicine!"). Try to stay cool when discussing asthma. Instead of preaching, try to engage your teen in some problem solving by asking brief questions such as, "What will happen if your asthma kicks up when you're in school?"

Rather than doling out ready-made solutions, ask your teenager to come up with some answers himself. You might say something like, "What can I do to help without being a nag?" Or, "I know that having asthma can be a daily hassle, as well as life threatening. It's important for me to know you're doing everything you can to keep it under control. That's why I remind you to take your controller medicines. But I want you to tell me *how* you want me to remind you." Or ask him to suggest some subtle prompts that serve as reminders for taking medicine—but don't let these prompts turn into nagging, and don't embarrass him with reminders in front of his friends. If you encourage a teenager to come up with his own solutions, he will be more motivated to follow through because he has had some active input.

Action

The third step—action—simply takes motivation one step further. Once a teenager is motivated to take more control and responsibility, she needs to know what to do—what precise action to take. That means learning symptom recognition, how to prevent symptoms, and what to do if a flare occurs. She should be encouraged to take note of when she coughs, wheezes, or experiences labored breathing or chest tightness. Ask her to think about how these symptoms affect her daily life—for example, coughing while watching a movie with friends or needing to stop playing a sport because of shortness of breath. Be sure she understands her asthma management plan and how to use it.

Another part of the "action" phase involves getting her to choose the time that she takes controller medicines. It often helps to have the therapy linked to an established daily behavior, such as getting in and out of bed or brushing teeth. Teens can also take on the responsibility of keeping track of the medicine supply and ordering refills when appropriate.

Each teenager will progress through this three-step process at a different pace, and it is important to provide support and reassurance while reinforcing the importance of adherence and asthma control.

SPECIAL CONSIDERATIONS

Three special considerations affect teenagers with asthma. The first is exercise-induced asthma, as discussed in chapter 11. During the teenage years, this issue may have a significant impact on the development of future exercise habits. In other words, if exercise triggers asthma symptoms, they can and should be controlled so that a teen with asthma is able to exercise and enjoy physical activities and sports as much as any other adolescent. It should not be an excuse to sit on the sidelines, which could lead to an unnecessarily sedentary life as an adult. The time to establish regular exercise as a healthy lifelong habit is now.

Teenagers with asthma should be carefully monitored for any symptoms that occur while exercising. If the symptoms are preventing participation in athletic activities, the therapy probably needs to be changed so the symptoms are better controlled. This may mean changing the medicines or adding medicines before exercise or sports activities. Ask your physician or nurse practitioner about your teen's specific situation.

A second consideration is smoking. Teenagers should receive counseling about exposure to tobacco smoke. Because smoking usually starts during adolescence, it is very important for teens with asthma to realize the "double risks" of tobacco use: (1) it makes the asthma more difficult or impossible to control, and (2) it increases long-term risks, such as emphysema, lung cancer, and heart disease. Though it's often overlooked, teenagers should also understand the importance of avoiding secondhand smoke from their friends who use tobacco.

The third consideration affects girls. Asthma can be especially bad for females entering adolescence. For reasons that are poorly understood, girls experiencing hormonal changes often encounter worsening asthma symptoms. In fact, puberty and adolescence are a peak time for asthma diagnosis in young women. It is not unusual for girls in their teens to be diagnosed with asthma for the first time, and adolescent girls with asthma often require an increase in their controller medicines.

For a teenager with asthma, the formidable period of adolescence can be more challenging than for teens without chronic diseases. Parents and health care professionals need to be patient and understanding and tailor their approach to each individual adolescent on the journey into adulthood. If adults support teenagers in becoming more mature and responsible for managing their disease, they can help young people enjoy the pleasures of adolescence with fewer symptoms and greater control.

14

Asthma Away from Home

Families are spending more and more time away from home. Infants and toddlers leave the house for day care. Older children and teens are busy with school, sports, and after-school activities. On weekends and vacations, families pack up for trips to relatives' homes, campsites, the beach, Disney World. . . . Everyone's on the go.

Children with a chronic condition like asthma should not be kept at home or restricted from any activity that other children enjoy. They should be able to go to school and camp and go on sleepovers, field trips, and family vacations. Yet parents need to be prepared for the unexpected when children with asthma are away from home. Even if your child's asthma is well controlled and she has no symptoms, it's best to plan ahead, use common sense, and be prepared so that experiences away from home will be enjoyable for your child and stress-free for you. In this chapter, you can walk through various away-from-home settings and consider how to manage your child's asthma effectively in each one.

AT DAY CARE AND SCHOOL

Kia's asthma was diagnosed when she was a year old, only a few months after she started attending a day care program. Her parents gave copies of her asthma management plan to the day care director and Kia's teacher. They reviewed the plan to be certain that everyone could recognize symptoms and give Kia quick-relief medicine when necessary. At home, her parents gave her controller medicine each morning and evening. Except when triggered by occasional colds—which seem to make perpetual rounds of day care centers—Kia's asthma was well controlled for the four years she attended day care. When she began elementary school, her parents again made her teachers and other school personnel aware of her asthma, gave them copies of her management plan, and made sure they understood how to implement it.

By the time Kia started middle school, her asthma was so well controlled that her parents let down their guard. Kia was now old enough to recognize symptoms herself, and she always carried a quick-relief inhaler and spacer in her backpack. Her parents didn't bother to contact the middle school personnel about her asthma. But after a few months in middle school, which was an older building, Kia's symptoms appeared more frequently. She still used a controller medicine at home, but her parents noticed that she was coughing more at night and often seemed short of breath.

With a little gentle prodding, her parents discovered that Kia had been using her quick-relief medicine much more often. They took her to the doctor who did a spirometry breathing test, reviewed the technique for administering her metered dose inhaler and spacer, and wrote new prescriptions with refills. In the end, they agreed that Kia's recent problems were probably related to triggers at school.

Her parents called the school nurse and told her of Kia's condition. They said they would send in a copy of Kia's asthma management plan and asked the nurse to review it with Kia's teachers. The nurse said she was happy to cooperate and mentioned, almost as an aside, that since she had started working at this middle school a few years ago, she was seeing a lot more students with asthma.

Kia's story had a happy ending. The school nurse and her teachers kept an eye on her, watched for symptoms, and quietly reminded Kia when to use her inhaler and spacer without making a big deal of it or drawing attention to her. More importantly, the school nurse took the lead in alerting the principal and faculty to the growing incidence of asthma at their school. By the end of the year, the old building had been thoroughly cleaned—air ducts, vents, radiators, shelves, ceiling tiles. As a school community, the PTA and staff made it a priority to be better informed about asthma and to keep triggers to a minimum.

One of the primary goals of successful asthma control is for children to be able to attend and participate in all day care and school activities. Since parents cannot guarantee this goal entirely on their own, the best way to achieve it is to work cooperatively with school and day care personnel. Some suggestions for doing that include:

- At the beginning of each school year, contact your child's teacher, school nurse, and any other personnel who are in contact with your child and inform them that she has asthma. (Include gym teachers and coaches; see chapter 11 for more about asthma, sports, and exercise.)

- Provide written instructions for your child's medicines and devices (nebulizer, MDI/spacer, DPI, or peak flow meter) to make sure your child doesn't miss any doses of medicine.

- Ask your child's doctor or nurse practitioner to fill out the necessary paperwork well ahead of time so your child won't miss any doses of medicine.

- Fill out school forms at the start of every school year. If your child's school has it own form with instructions for administering medicine, fill it out completely and be sure that your physician completes and signs the appropriate part. Attach a copy of your child's asthma management plan to the forms.

- When a permission slip comes home for a class trip to a zoo, farm, or other destination where your child might encounter asthma triggers, attach a note to remind the teacher to look over your child's asthma management plan and take along contact information (for you and your child's doctor or nurse practitioner) in the event a flare occurs.

School Policies on Medicines

Some schools don't have a full-time school nurse, so ask the principal or your child's teacher who will be responsible for giving medicine when the nurse is not in school. Policies about children carrying and taking their own medicine vary, depending on state and school regulations, so it's important to learn your local policies and plan ahead before a crisis arises.

The use of medicine in school can be controversial. Health experts agree that children with asthma should have ready, easy access to their quick-relief medicines. But medicine is included in many schools' "zero tolerance" drug policies, so students are not permitted to keep medicine in their pockets, bookbags, or lockers. Although it is very rare, prohibiting students from carrying medicine with them has had fatal results. The worst possible result, reported by the *New York Times* in 2002, was the death of a child who developed asthma symptoms in school but had not been allowed to carry his quick-relief medicine with him. By the time he received any medicine, it was too late.

This rare tragedy highlights the need for parents to be proactive and educate not only their child's teachers but also school administrators about asthma and its consequences. Parents can make a difference by becoming involved when school boards make policies that could be a matter of life and death.

Triggers at School

The risk of exposure to triggers is another important consideration at day care or school. You may have done everything necessary to remove asthma triggers from your home, but your child spends six or more hours each day in school or day care. Take a look around that environment. In Kia's old middle school building, triggers were easy to spot. But most schools—whether the building is new or old—contain a slew of asthma triggers: dust in carpeting or from chalk; class pets (those cute gerbils, hamsters, and rabbits); cockroaches; strong odors and chemicals used in science, art, or other classes and for cleaning the school; and smoke. Although smoking should be banned in schools, it still occurs.

As an individual parent, you can influence some positive changes if you discuss asthma triggers with school personnel. You can request that animals be removed from the classroom and moved elsewhere. If your child is bothered by chalk dust, he could be seated farther away from the blackboard. If he naps at day care or school, provide his own pillow with a protective covering. Suggest to the school principal that cockroaches are reduced by thorough cleaning, especially in the kitchen and cafeteria areas and through regular exterminating treatments and use of traps. Exterminating, cleaning with chemicals, or maintaining the grounds (mowing the grass or playing fields) should be done before or after school hours.

If you don't want to stand out as a solitary critic, find other parents of children with asthma and approach school administrators as a small group to make these recommendations. At home, you work hard to keep your child's asthma under control, so don't hesitate to ask others to make a collective effort to protect all children with asthma from triggers at day care and school. Children shouldn't miss school because of this disease. They should be able to pay attention to their schoolwork, participate in all activities, and rarely need to take quick-relief medicine if triggers are eliminated.

SLEEPOVERS

Jasmine was doing well when she was invited to sleep over at her friend Katelynn's home. Jasmine's mother didn't know that Katelynn had a dog and a cat. At the time of the sleepover, Jasmine's asthma was under good control. She was doing so well, in fact, that her mom forgot to tell Katelynn's parents about her asthma and her allergy to dogs and cats.

Soon after arriving at Katelynn's, Jasmine developed a stuffed-up, runny nose and began sneezing. With three other children visiting for the evening, Katelynn's mother didn't think much about it. She noticed that Jasmine was sneezing quite a bit, but she knew that several school friends had been passing colds around that week.

During the night, Jasmine coughed and wheezed so much that she woke herself up. She knew she was starting to have an asthma flare and called home. Her dad came and picked her up in the middle of the night. As soon as they got home, they started her asthma management plan and she improved quickly. But it was an embarrassing lesson for Jasmine—and a serious one for her parents. They decided that the next time she was invited to a party or a friend's home, they would talk to the host family about possible triggers in their home. They would also give Jasmine medicine before going to the friend's house, talk about possibly having the party at another location away from pets or other triggers, and would send medicine with a copy of her asthma management plan with her.

Children with asthma want to sleep over at friends' homes just like other children. In general, parents have to decide if the environment will be okay for them. Children shouldn't be in a position of feeling sick but too embarrassed to tell anyone—a recipe for a serious flare. Some general guidelines include:

- The sleepover site should be "tobacco smoke free" and have no pets if your child is allergic to them.

- It will probably not be dust free, but you can send along a sleeping pallet (something as simple as a thin blanket or plastic sheet) in addition to her sleeping bag to create a barrier between your child and the carpet.

- Once you decide that she is allowed to sleep over, contact the adult in charge regardless of what your child says. Let your child know that this adult needs to be aware of how to help her if she starts having problems.

- Talk to your child about possible activities that may happen at the sleepover (like pillow fights that would produce clouds of dust). Also talk about where she would feel comfortable taking her medicines and when would be the best time. Encourage her to be open with her friends about having asthma.

- Make a pouch with her quick-relief medicines, her control medicines, and her asthma management plan.

- If it's her first time staying at a new place, take the time to review the plan with the adult in charge. As your child gets older, she should be able to take on more responsibility to the point where she can manage her medicines independently. Let her know that ultimately the goal is for her to take control of her asthma.

CAMP

Dylan went to camp for the first time last summer. His parents did everything right. They organized all his medicines, sent an extra spacer, got him a special backpack to hold his medicines for day outings, and gave the camp nurse a copy of his asthma management plan. So what could possibly go wrong?

Dylan loved camp. He made new friends in his bunk, learned to swim, and showed no asthma symptoms—until the third week of camp, when his group went horseback riding. Dylan excitedly climbed on his horse and within a few minutes his eyes started to itch and water. His nose got congested, and he started sneezing. An alert counselor took him back to the infirmary where the camp nurse treated his allergic reaction, gave him a dose of albuterol, and Dylan quickly improved. The nurse then called Dylan's parents to notify them of his allergic reaction to the horse, report that he was fine again, and suggested that they have him evaluated by an allergist.

Everything worked smoothly for Dylan in this case, but his parents learned that they must make sure they know ahead of time how medical emergencies will be handled. If you're planning to send your child to day or overnight camp, ask about the camp's policies and procedures for emergencies and what medical personnel will be available to handle them.

WHENEVER SOMEONE ELSE IS IN CHARGE

Common sense and planning are essential when children with asthma go away from home without a parent. You need to communicate with anyone who will be taking care of your child. This includes relatives, baby-sitters, day care personnel, teachers, coaches, school nurses, friends' parents, camp counselors, and other adults who will be responsible when you aren't with your child. Keep in mind that many people don't have an accurate understanding of asthma. A lot of old myths about asthma are floating around that people still believe are true (common myths are listed in Resources).

Here is a basic list of what other adults need to know:

- Names of your child's medicines
- When to give them (daily and/or when symptoms occur)
- How to give the medicine
- What symptoms indicate a problem
- What to expect from the medicine (for example, they shouldn't expect immediate relief from a long-term controller medicine but should from a quick-relief medicine)
- What to do if the child doesn't improve or gets worse after taking a quick-relief medicine
- Who to call in an emergency (parents' work/cellular numbers, backup person if parents aren't reachable, child's physician, ambulance, nearest hospital)

Much of the above will be listed in your child's written asthma management plan, a copy of which should be given to those who are caring for your child.

If you don't know the answers to all these points, sit down with your child's physician or nurse practitioner and come up with a list together. Request prescriptions that you need now or in the near future, especially if you're planning a trip. Do you need an extra spacer, inhaler, or nebulizer that will stay at day care, school, camp, or Grandma's house? It's just a matter of being prepared.

TRAVELING WITH A CHILD WHO HAS ASTHMA

> Mindy is a toddler with mild persistent asthma. She had never been hospitalized or treated in the emergency room. On a family trip to Florida, she ended up in the emergency room with an asthma attack. This took her parents totally by surprise because her asthma had always been under control. She was treated at a local hospital emergency room that did not specialize in pediatrics. Mindy did well, but this little detour in the family vacation certainly frightened her parents.

When planning any trip, you map out a route and make reservations. When you pack for a trip, you consider where you are going, how you will be getting there, how long you will be away, and what the weather will be like. You don't just randomly throw things into a suitcase. You select the right type of clothes and accessories (such as sunscreen), make sure they are in good condition, and pack them so you will be able to get to them when you need them.

Asthma never takes a vacation, so asthma therapy shouldn't either. Planning ahead to keep asthma under control during travel requires similar planning. When you're prepared, there should be no interruption in therapy during travel. Being prepared means figuring out in advance where you can get expert treatment if your child develops an asthma flare, both along the way and at your destination. Think about the environment you will be visiting. Is it dry, dusty, damp? Could there be potential triggers to which your child isn't normally exposed? Remember that your child may seem fine, but in an environment away from home, you never know what triggers your child might encounter.

Your daily schedule on a trip will probably differ from routines at home, so figure out when asthma treatments can be realistically given during the trip, make a schedule, and stick to it. If you miss a dose or two, your child could possibly develop a flare, and that would put a damper on your plans.

Some other travel tips are:

- Make sure you have a full supply of controller and quick-relief medicines, as well as their necessary delivery devices. A vacation is not the time to let your teenager use his inhaler without the spacer just so he doesn't have to pack it.

- Bring contact information for your child's physician or nurse practitioner, and pharmacy.

- Be sure to take along a copy of your child's asthma management plan.

- If you are planning a car trip that will take more than a few hours, plan treatment stops along the way. It is safer and more efficient to give medicine—especially inhaled medicine—when the car is stopped so you can give your full attention to the treatment.

- Before you leave home, identify hospitals at your destination where you can go for urgent care, just in case.

Medicine When Traveling

Before packing asthma medicines for a trip, keep these suggestions in mind:

- Take extra medicine. Pack one and a half times what you think you'll need for the number of days you'll be away in case you are delayed, the trip is extended, or you have to use more medicine than usual because your child experiences an asthma flare.

- All medicines should travel in appropriate containers. Keep them in the containers they came in from the pharmacy. All the necessary information should be on the pharmacy label. Labels should show the child's name, medicine name, dose, name of the prescriber, and the medicine's strength. Many parents know the name of their child's medicine but not its strength; this can cause problems because many medicines come in multiple strengths.

- Pack medicines so you'll have immediate access to them at any time during the trip. They should be packed so that they're protected from getting wet or from extreme temperatures. When traveling by car, keep medicines up front in the passenger area, not in the trunk or glove compartment, which can become too warm. On a plane, keep medicines with you in a carry-on bag. Do not pack them in a suitcase that will be checked and stowed in the baggage compartment. It is more likely to get lost and could be exposed to temperature extremes.

- Have quick-relief medicine available at all times. Don't leave it behind at the hotel when you go out for the day.

If your child takes medicine by nebulizer, you may want to consider obtaining a portable nebulizer, which is usually smaller than a regular nebulizer and runs on batteries or a car cigarette lighter (DC power) rather than plugging a cord into an electrical outlet. A portable nebulizer is convenient for travel, but it is usually less powerful than a regular nebulizer, so treatments may take longer. And some portable nebulizers do not put out the proper medicine-particle-size mist. (Only certain size particles can go down into the small airways.)

Another consideration is the fact that many health insurers will not cover the cost of a second nebulizer, let alone a portable one that is more expensive. If you decide to get one, you may have to pay for it out-of-pocket. Another option you might want to discuss with your child's physician or nurse practitioner is switching from a nebulizer to MDIs with a spacer, as long as the medicine your child takes is available in that form and you learn how to use the device properly ahead of time. These devices can be used successfully even in infants, as long as they're used with a face mask.

If you bring a nebulizer on a plane trip, you will probably need to check it with luggage rather than carry it on board with you. Since luggage is sometimes lost, it is a good idea to identify an equipment company near your destination that will rent a nebulizer for the length of your stay just in case.

Special Considerations for Flying

Two special circumstances apply to airplane travel and asthma. First, air inside a plane cabin is recycled. Second, air in a plane is thinner, or has less oxygen. If your child's asthma is not under control before getting on the plane, your child may have increased symptoms. Consider postponing travel if your child is having a difficult-to-control flare. Planes are diverted to the nearest airport only in a life-or-death medical emergency, but otherwise they continue to the planned destination. If your child has a flare that becomes worse on board, the flight will seem painfully long for everyone involved. The best advice is to get your child's flare under control before you fly.

Going Abroad

International travel makes planning even more complicated. These trips absolutely require that all medicines be properly labeled. Make sure that you take along enough medicine to last the entire trip because the exact same medicine may not be available in the country you're visiting. You should also keep a copy of your child's asthma management plan with the medicine.

Plug adapters may also be needed if you are going to use a nebulizer because electrical outlets abroad may differ from those in the United States. Adapters for different countries are available where luggage is sold. If you're visiting a country where you don't speak the language, make sure that you identify hospitals in advance.

Asthma and its treatment should not be any more burdensome while traveling than it is at home if you use common sense, plan ahead, and prepare to have a safe and enjoyable trip. Bon voyage!

15

Asthma in Your Community

A s a parent, your first concern is your own child. Previous chapters have focused on understanding your child's asthma and controlling and treating it as effectively as possible. But you may want to reach beyond your child's individual situation to help families and others in your community bring the growing incidence of childhood asthma under control. It's the old tried-and-true "strength in numbers" strategy: by working together, groups of people can attack a problem more successfully than a single individual. Toward that goal, this chapter describes a model program that has been working successfully in our own neighborhood under the sponsorship of The Children's Hospital of Philadelphia. You may want to consider using this model to develop a similar approach in your own community.

THE PHILADELPHIA COMMUNITY ASTHMA PREVENTION PROGRAM

Many studies have shown that two factors are essential to improve the quality of life of people with asthma: increasing their knowledge of the disease and improving their environment. The Philadelphia Community Asthma Prevention Program (CAPP) was established in 1997 to address these issues in the West Philadelphia community. Remarkably successful in only a few years, it is being replicated in North Philadelphia as well.

As a community-based program, CAPP provides a comprehensive, community-based program to promote an optimal learning environment for asthma education. CAPP's specific goals include educating children and families to control exposure to asthma triggers, form asthma management plans, monitor lung function, and improve self-management behavior. It also trains members of the community to become asthma educators and partners with families to improve the quality of life for children with asthma. To these ends, CAPP developed three main components: community education classes, a train-the-trainer program, and a home visitor program.

Community Education Classes

Classes for both children and adults are taught in small groups with discussions led by peer educators. CAPP's community asthma education classes are held in community centers, schools, churches, and day care centers. In CAPP's first four years, they reached over 1,600 parents and children with asthma.

Parents and children are taught simultaneously in separate classes. Classes are open to the entire community and are advertised in local newspapers, Laundromats, libraries, and doctors' offices. Conducted in one-hour sessions, classes run once a week for five weeks. Each class addresses a different aspect of asthma. Children's classes are geared toward five-year-olds and older and are taught by trained teenage peer educators. Trained parent peers teach parents' classes. The curriculum used for the program is the "You Can Control Asthma" curriculum developed by Georgetown University and written for low-literacy audiences (fifth-grade reading level). This curriculum is widely available and can be ordered from The Asthma and Allergy Foundation of America (see Resources, page 234).

In the first class, participants discuss how asthma affects the body. During week two, they discover what asthma triggers are and learn techniques to avoid them. The most popular class occurs in the third week when participants are instructed to bring in their medicines and discuss their proper use; asthma devices, such as inhalers and spacers, are also demonstrated. The fourth week's class focuses on the peak flow meter and asthma management plan based on the medicines prescribed by their physicians. Week five's class concludes with a discussion of family and school issues. More than 75 percent of participants who enroll in the classes complete the five-week class series. Below is a summary of the five sessions.

Session 1: Introduction to CAPP	What is asthma and why does my child have it? In this session we will explain how asthma affects your child's body.
Session 2: Triggers of Asthma and Prevention Techniques	We will talk about different things in the environment that trigger asthma. We will teach you how to avoid these triggers and to prevent an asthma attack from starting.
Session 3: Medicines and Devices	We will explain the differences in the medicines how they work to keep asthma symptoms from starting, and how they calm the symptoms once they begin. We will talk about the purpose of the devices, the proper way to use them, and how to take care of them.
Session 4: Asthma Management Plan	We will talk about using your peak flow meter and developing a management plan for your child. This will give you the information that you need to treat asthma symptoms early. You're going to feel really in control after this session!
Session 5: School and Family Issues	We will discuss ways to help your teacher and school nurse deal with your child's asthma. We will also look at how asthma affects the family as a whole. We will discuss what your family can do to relieve stress, yet at the same time be supportive to your child.

After the five classes, participants showed an improved awareness of what causes asthma, how to control it, and of parental perception of quality of life. This improvement was demonstrated by comparing scores on tests they took before starting the CAPP series and after they completed it. And they didn't forget what they learned. Parents retained both knowledge and skills for twelve months, according to follow-up study. Children also showed ongoing improvement: of those who didn't use a spacer or peak flow meters prior to the classes, 78 percent were using spacers within a year after the classes and 52 percent were using peak flow meters.

Train-the-Trainer

The second component of CAPP—the train-the-trainer sessions—helps key people in the community learn how to provide asthma education. CAPP identifies highly motivated parents in the community classes and trains them to be class teachers or parent educators. Under the supervision of a CAPP coordinator, trained parents initially coteach and eventually graduate to become lead teacher of other classes. This key component has been so successful that parent asthma educators currently teach all of CAPP's community classes.

CAPP has also trained primary care physicians, nurse practitioners, and office staff within the community. Since its start in 1997, CAPP has trained 15 parent facilitators and 20 peer educators, 60 school nurses, and 130 physicians and physicians-in-training. A training manual for parent educators and school nurses was written by CAPP staff and includes information on asthma, adult learning theory and techniques, practice teaching materials, and strategies for teaching low-literacy audiences.

The Home Visitor Program

The third component of CAPP, the Home Intervention Program, was developed to determine if comprehensive, low-cost, scientifically proven interventions to remove common indoor triggers (dust, tobacco smoke pollution, molds, cockroaches, and animal dander) would improve the quality of life for people with persistent asthma.

Home Visits Summary

Visit	Education	Intervention
First	Project explained to family	Consent form signed. Home assessment completed.
Second	Asthma as a disease Signs and symptoms of an asthma attack Review of medicines in home	Roach and mice bait given with instructions on proper use. Other methods of pest control discussed.
Third	Common indoor asthma triggers Avoidance techniques	Dusters and mattress and pillow covers given with instructions for use. Demonstration of the use of mattress and pillow covers. Carpet removal or vacuum bags given.
Fourth	In-depth review of asthma medicines and devices	Cockroach and pet dander avoidance techniques. Sponge and buckets given. Demonstration on proper method to wash baseboards.
Fifth	Asthma Management Plan	Trash bags, shades, and shade brackets given.

Program participants receive resources and support to remove common indoor asthma triggers from the child's bedroom at different stages over a twelve-month period. Families receive regular visits from home visitors who are members of the community trained to provide education one-on-one to parents and children and to help adjust the environment to reduce asthma triggers. Families are asked to keep a diary to record asthma symptoms and use of medicines.

This project has successfully and significantly reduced carpeting, cockroaches, rodents, and tobacco smoke pollution in the homes of children with asthma. In-home classes and environmental intervention have been completed in more than 280 homes. With younger children, this intervention has resulted in fewer emergency room visits and hospitalizations. Participants' nighttime and daytime asthma symptoms have been reduced overall.

CAPP owes its success to the principles of peer education, home intervention, and equipping community members to become asthma champions. CAPP is a model for community-based interventions to improve the lives of children with asthma. We hope the children in your community can also benefit from such a program.

16

Asthma and the
Health Care System

E arlier chapters have offered information about understanding, controlling, and treating your child's asthma. But as parents of children
with chronic diseases know all too well, there's more to caring for a
child than giving medicine and getting to doctors' appointments. There's
also a sea of bureaucracy—the "health care system" of insurance forms,
referrals, specialists, bills, copays, deductibles, prescriptions, medical
devices. . . .

Caring for a child with asthma may sometimes feel like a journey
across unfamiliar waters. Your primary care provider's office may serve
as a home base, but other important ports of call may include subspe-
cialists, visiting nurses, medical supply companies, and other providers.
Unfortunately, the coordinates for this journey are not mapped out
clearly for you in advance. Our health care system is complex and ever
changing. Financial and bureaucratic obstacles still prevent many children from receiving the care they need.

Social workers can help families work through these challenges. You
are fortunate if a social worker is playing an active role on your child's
team. If not, an experienced social worker has contributed information

to this chapter that will give you insight into successfully navigating the health care system. You can use this information to help create a team that includes your child's doctor and other health care professionals. Parents should not have to carry the burden alone.

Private Health Insurance

Asthma care and medicines are expensive, and obtaining the right health insurance is an important first step in accessing the health care system. Recent changes in the law provide the opportunity for virtually every child in every state to qualify for some form of health insurance. The rules and steps involved are complex, however, and may leave many gaps in the care that is provided. Gone are the days when parents could assume that any type of health insurance would pay for all the care that a child with asthma requires.

If your child has private insurance through your employer, you need to explore what it covers. Inpatient (in-hospital) and outpatient (office) benefits may be treated differently and may include copays and deductibles that come out of your pocket before the insurance coverage starts to pay. Some insurance plans provide full payment only to providers who are within the plan's own "network." If this is the case, it's important to be sure that the network includes your child's primary care doctor or pediatrician, nurse practitioner, and other health care professionals. A referral from your primary care provider may be needed for the insurance plan to cover fully any specialists, such as allergy or pulmonary doctors.

With the increasing costs of medicines, most insurance companies have cut back on prescription plans. Many plans include copays, prior authorization, or require the use of a mail-order prescription company. Generic forms of some asthma medicines are available and may result in lower costs if prescribed by your doctor or nurse practitioner. By and large, generic drugs for asthma work just as well as name brands.

If your insurance does not cover prescriptions, there are other options to consider. Some pharmaceutical companies offer assistance plans;

information can be obtained by contacting the individual company directly. Clinical research trials also will sometimes cover the cost of medicines. Information about clinical trials can be obtained through drug companies, your physician, or through an Internet site set up by the National Institutes of Health (www.ClinicalTrials.gov). Durable medical equipment, such as nebulizers and other home care needs, are covered differently by insurance plans. Some forms of equipment, such as spacers, can be ordered at low cost from organizations such as the Allergy & Asthma Network: Mothers of Asthmatics (www.aanma.org or 1-800-878-4403).

PUBLIC INSURANCE

If you do not have private insurance, several options are available for public insurance. These programs use funds from the federal government but are organized differently in each state. You can learn the specific rules for your area by calling your local county Board of Assistance. Medical Assistance (also known as Medicaid) offers coverage to children under the age of nineteen based on income, residency, and other requirements. Many state Medicaid programs involve managed care plans that have rules about specialty care similar to private insurance plans.

In 1997, the federal government established the Children's Health Insurance Program (CHIP) to expand the availability of health insurance coverage to working families beyond what Medicaid provides. The federal government funds the states to help pay for this program. Since the program is administered by each state, the specific rules may vary in your area. In most states, children from a family of four, with earnings up to $34,100 per year (in 2002), are eligible. More information about the CHIP program can be obtained by calling 1-877-KIDS-NOW.

Some children with chronic diseases like asthma may be eligible for Supplemental Security Income (SSI) as determined by financial and medical criteria. There are strict guidelines, but an eligible child may receive cash assistance as well as medical insurance. Information about SSI can be obtained through the Social Security Administration at 1-800-772-1213 or through your local Social Security office.

PRIMARY CARE

Every child should have a primary care provider for well-child checkups and immunizations. With a chronic disease like asthma, it is particularly important to see consistently the same physician, nurse practitioner, or other professional over time so the primary care provider can get to know your child well. This primary care provider will play the lead role in assessing your child's asthma, prescribing medicines, and making referrals for other services or specialty care if needed.

Primary care providers differ in many ways, including their training background (for example: family medicine, pediatrics, and nurse practitioner programs), the structure of their offices (private office, hospital, or public clinic), and the size of their practice (a single provider or a large group).

Choosing a primary care provider is a personal decision, but several factors are important to consider when your child has asthma.

- **Experience with young asthma patients:** The provider should be familiar with treating asthma in the pediatric age range. Children have many unique needs that require a treatment approach different from that for adults.

- **Access:** Since asthma flares can occur at unpredictable times, you should always be able to reach someone for advice. Many offices are open for evening and weekend hours, which can be very convenient for working parents.

- **Support systems:** Last but certainly not least, the other staff and support services are important. A friendly, accessible office staff and a well-organized system for teaching about asthma, refilling prescriptions, and following through on patients' needs can add a great deal to your child's care. Some offices may have specifically trained staff, such as social workers or case managers, available to help with obtaining services. A team approach to primary care has the most to offer.

SPECIALTY CARE

Specialty care for asthma can be confusing because each type of provider may have a different focus. Pediatric allergists specialize in the reactions of the immune system to common environmental allergens, such as pollens, dust mites, or pet dander, that can play a key role in asthma. Allergists use skin tests to detect allergies and may, in some cases, treat allergies by giving repeated small doses of the allergen (see chapter 3). Pediatric pulmonary medicine physicians (also known as pulmonologists) specialize in lung diseases in children. These physicians perform lung function tests and procedures such as bronchoscopy, where a small camera is used to look inside the lung. Both allergists and pulmonologists treat asthma with the conventional medicines that have been described in this book. In specific cases, however, they may have a somewhat different approach to diagnosis and management of asthma.

Whether your child needs to see a specialist is an individual question to be discussed with your primary care provider. In most cases, mild asthma can be managed successfully by your regular physician or pediatrician. But a specialist can be very helpful if your child does not seem to be responding well to treatment or if your primary care provider has specific concerns and suggests that further testing may be needed. Beyond having added experience and training, specialists usually schedule extra time to delve into the specifics of more difficult cases. Since they focus on asthma, they may also have educational material, support staff, and other resources that can be very useful to you and your child.

Visiting a specialist may pose some potential problems. With more than one provider now treating your child, there is the potential for confusion and miscommunication. It's important to make sure that information flows well between the specialist and your primary care provider, who will continue to prescribe your child's medicines and see your child for acute illnesses.

Specialty care is expensive and can pose financial hardship if not covered by insurance, so it's important to make sure that referrals and other needed forms are completed before seeing a specialist.

ASTHMA CARE IN THE HOME

Home care is a growing area of medicine that is very applicable to asthma. In addition to teaching about asthma in the comfort of a child's usual setting, home care staff can check asthma equipment, such as nebulizers, and assess the condition of the home. Eliminating allergens and improving the air quality of a home can dramatically improve asthma symptoms for some children, as discussed in chapter 10. Some health insurers recognize the value of home visits and may provide these services in selected cases. If you feel that a home visit would be helpful for your child, discuss this possibility with your primary care provider.

MAKING THE SYSTEM WORK FOR YOUR CHILD

Many different types of health services are available for children with asthma. Most children will do well with simple interventions, but if your child is having difficulty, it is important to ask about what else can be done. Obtaining additional services may require approvals from your primary care provider or insurance company. Well-run insurance companies have recognized that although these services cost money, in the long run they may prevent expensive emergency visits and hospital care.

Since asthma is such a common condition, many insurance companies have developed asthma programs that attempt to identify children who are not doing well and link them with services such as home nursing visits, asthma education classes and printed materials, and asthma specialists. A case manager, often a nurse or social worker with experience in asthma, may be assigned to your child to help make sure that appropriate services are provided. You may want to ask your insurance company about the availability of such a person. If not, don't hesitate to advocate for your child and take on this role with the help of your primary care provider.

Although caring for a child with asthma can be a daunting journey, many supports and services are available to help families along the way. Viewing asthma care as a team approach—your family, your primary care doctor, nurse practitioner, office staff, and others as needed—will help make treating asthma smooth sailing for your child.

Glossary of Common Asthma-Related Terms

airways   Passages throughout the respiratory system for inhaling and exhaling air into and out of the lungs: the nose, windpipe (trachea), and bronchial tubes. Airways are lined with mucus that traps irritating particles (like dust and smoke) and tiny hairs that sweep up these particles and keep them from being inhaled deeper into the lungs. People with asthma have sensitive airways.

albuterol   Generic name for a class of medicines that are commonly used, short-acting bronchodilators for quick relief of symptoms (like wheezing and shortness of breath); typically administered by an aerosol metered dose inhaler (MDI) with a spacer. Also available in pill or liquid form (an oral preparation as syrup) or as a liquid for a nebulizer that mixes it into a mist for inhalation; common brand names: Proventil, Ventolin, and Xopenex (levalbuterol); used on an as-needed basis and not as a preventive or controller medicine.

allergen   Any substance that can cause an allergic reaction; typical examples are pollen, dust, pet dander.

allergist   A physician trained to diagnose and treat allergic disorders affecting especially the eyes, nose, throat, lungs, skin, intestinal tract, as well as reaction to foods, drugs, and insects; also trained in immune deficiency disorders.

allergy   Hypersensitivity to certain irritating substances (allergens).

alveoli   Pockets of tiny air sacs that split off from bronchioles within each lung. Within alveoli, oxygen from inhaled air is absorbed into the bloodstream in exchange for carbon dioxide waste, which is exhaled. The adult lung has 300 million alveoli.

antihistamine   Medicine that treats allergies by neutralizing histamine, which causes itch, mucus production, and some swelling in areas where it is released (examples: Benadryl, Claritin, Zyrtec).

anti-inflammatory medicines   A class of medicines that reduce airway swelling and help prevent asthma flares; these controller medicines should be used regularly whether or not a child is experiencing asthma symptoms.

asthma   A chronic respiratory disease in which sensitive airways become inflamed, narrow, and obstructed when muscles surrounding them tighten and squeeze them, and excessive mucus is produced; resulting symptoms include shortness of breath, chest tightness, wheezing, coughing.

bronchus (singular), bronchi (plural)   The main airways branching off from the trachea (windpipe) to each lung.

bronchioles   Smaller tubes or airways branching off from the bronchi; the lungs have tens of thousands of bronchioles.

bronchodilator   Medicine that opens up—or dilates—the airways by relaxing the smooth muscles around the airway walls; can be administered by inhaler or nebulizer; often used to prevent exercise-induced asthma symptoms when used fifteen to thirty minutes before exercise or sports activity.

bronchospasm   Squeezing or tightening of the muscles surrounding the airways, which obstructs them and makes breathing difficult.

controller medicines   A class of medicines that provide long-term control of asthma, usually by decreasing airway inflammation and its symptoms; given regularly to prevent symptoms and flares; not for immediate relief of symptoms or flares.

corticosteroids   A class of medicines that decrease inflammation; inhaled corticosteroids (ICS) are considered the most effective controller medicine for people with persistent asthma; not for quick relief of symptoms. Used regularly, they make triggers less likely to cause symptoms; they take several days or weeks to have full effect; not the same as anabolic steroids used to build muscle. Topical corticosteroids (like hydrocortisone) are applied to the skin to treat atopic dermatitis (skin inflammation, redness, itching) caused by allergies.

dander   Flakes of skin or dried saliva from animals with fur or feathers. Materials derived from glands in the skin, saliva, urine, and blood adhere to the dander flakes; when people with allergies inhale bits of dander, they react to the allergens that the dander carries.

dry powder inhaler (DPI)   A device for delivering inhaled bronchodilator medicines deep into the lungs by the force of a rapid inspiration; requires a fast, deep breath; can typically be used by children over age four, but they need to be taught to use it correctly (examples: Serevent, Diskus, Advair, Foradil).

dust mites   Tiny, invisible bugs that live in carpets and fabrics. Dust mites eat human skin flakes; their droppings contain allergens that trigger allergic reactions in humans.

eczema, or atopic dermatitis   An allergic condition of the skin; symptoms include itching, dryness, redness or scaling; often triggered by allergens in the air or by foods; 40 percent of children with eczema may have varying degrees of asthma.

exercise-induced asthma   Symptoms caused by increased demands on the respiratory system by physical exertion. With exercise, breathing is deeper and faster; air in the lungs is cooler and drier than usual, which is believed to stimulate inflammatory cells in the airways; this in turn makes the airways swell or produce mucus. The cells also irritate and tighten muscles that encircle the airways. Chest tightness and shortness of breath appear about five minutes after exercise begins, with wheezing and coughing following. Exercise-induced asthma can be improved by using short-acting bronchodilators fifteen to thirty minutes before starting to exercise and by good everyday control of asthma.

flare   An episode or "attack" when asthma symptoms become worse and cause increased breathing difficulties, coughing, wheezing, chest tightness, or shortness of breath. Flares can be mild or severe; parents should know what to do when symptoms worsen into a flare.

gastroesophageal reflux disease (also called **acid reflux**)   A condition in which stomach contents and acid travel back up the esophagus; reflux causes asthma worsening by irritating the esophagus and triggering a reflex action, or directly increasing bronchospasm in the airways. Reflux doesn't create an asthmatic condition per se, but when present in someone with asthma, it can make asthma control more difficult.

inflammation   The reaction of tissues to irritants or injury, resulting in swelling, pain, redness, or heat. Normally, inflammation can be helpful to the body by clearing harmful materials (such as infection, foreign matter like a splinter, or even tumor cells). In allergic inflammation, the body reacts to an allergen. In the case of asthma, the lining of airways becomes inflamed.

inhaler   A small, handheld device used to deliver medicine into the lungs. Inhalers come in various forms: metered dose inhalers (MDIs) deliver precise amounts of medicine with each inhaled puff; MDIs should be used with spacers and require a slow deep breath. Dry powder inhalers deliver medicine as a fine, dry powder and require a quick deep breath.

leukotrienes   Natural substances produced by the body that cause muscles in the airways to contract and lung tissue to swell. The result—breathing difficulty—can be treated by **anti-leukotriene medicine** (nonsteroid controller medicine) that reduces swelling.

mast cell   Cells found throughout the body that react quickly to allergens. When someone with allergies comes in contact with an allergen like pollen or dust, the body makes more naturally occurring antibodies called IgE, which then attach to mast cells and set off an allergic reaction; the mast cells burst open and release a number of substances, including histamine, that causes redness, swelling, and itching.

mast cell stabilizers   A class of nonsteroid controller medicine that reduces the release of inflammation-causing chemicals from mast cells; available in inhaled and/or nebulized form (examples: Cromolyn, Nedocromil).

metered dose inhaler (MDI)   A delivery device that releases an exact, measured amount of asthma medicine from an aerosol canister each time a child inhales a puff.

nebulizer   The cup part of a machine that delivers asthma medicine in a fine mist that is inhaled through either a face mask or mouthpiece; an attached air compressor provides a stream of air to create the mist. Liquid medicine is placed in the nebulizer cup and converted into small droplets that remain in the mist long enough to be inhaled into the lungs.

peak flow meter   A small, inexpensive device that measures how fast air moves out of the child's lungs when a child exhales; it measures the **peak expiratory flow (PEF),** which is an indicator of airway size.

pulmonary function test (PFT)   Assessment of the lungs' capacity and function; measures the amount of air and how fast it is exhaled.

pulmonologist   A physician who specializes in respiratory (lung) conditions, including asthma.

quick-relief medicines   A group of medicines used to relieve asthma symptoms when they occur; not used for prevention or control of asthma; sometimes also called "rescue" medicines. Quick-relief medicines work as short-acting bronchodilators that open the airways by relaxing the muscles that surround them.

spacer   A device attached to a metered dose inhaler (MDI) that helps deliver inhaled asthma medicine deep into the lungs; acts as "a holding chamber" because it holds, or suspends, the medicine spray so that a child can inhale a slow, deep breath. Spacers (such as Aerochamber or Optichamber) are recommended because they help to reduce the amount of medicine that can stick in the mouth or throat or be swallowed when using an MDI.

spirometry   A special breathing test (also known as pulmonary function testing or PFT) that measures how blocked the airways are by the swelling and squeezing of asthma.

theophylline   A bronchodilator used as both controller and quick-relief medicine; available in syrup, pill, and injectable forms; does not have significant anti-inflammatory effects, so it became less popular as a preventive treatment when the role of inflammation in asthma was recognized.

trigger   Any irritant or allergen that produces symptoms; asthma triggers typically include viruses (colds and flu), environmental irritants (such as smoke, perfumes, and chemicals), and allergens (such as dust, pollen from grass and trees, pet dander, mold, dust mites, and insects like cockroaches). When asthma is not well controlled, other triggers may also include physical exercise, laughing, crying, or cold weather.

wheezing   One of the common symptoms of asthma; sounds like a high-pitched whistling; results from a narrowing of the airways that is caused by inflammation, tightening of muscles around airways, and excess mucus produced by the lungs. Not every patient with asthma will wheeze while having other symptoms. Wheezing can disappear when airways get very narrow—this is a sign of a serious flare.

Resources

T his book was intended to provide useful information to help parents and other adults understand asthma and the importance of controlling it by preventing symptoms and treating them quickly and appropriately when they arise. One read-through of this book, however, may not be enough because asthma is a chronic, ongoing disease. Undoubtedly times will arise when you may need to pull this book off the shelf and refer back to particular sections. To help you refresh your knowledge, we are providing the following resource material. We suggest that you reread it from time to time and not only in times of an asthma flare or crisis.

You are also encouraged to photocopy any of these pages and give them to others involved in the care of your child. You can use some of these tools, such as the Asthma Management Plan or School Management Plan in particular, as blank forms that you and your child's physician or nurse practitioner can fill in with specific information about your child's symptoms and treatment.

The Resources section includes:

- What Is Asthma?
- A Review of the Allergy-Asthma Connection
- Frequently Asked Questions about Asthma
- A Review of Asthma Medicines
- Asthma Medicines
- A Guide to Using Spacers
- A Guide to Using a Peak Flow Meter
- The Children's Hospital of Philadelphia's Asthma Management Plan
- Eliminating Asthma Triggers
- A School Management Plan
- How Asthma-Friendly Is Your School or Day Care Center?
- Famous People with Asthma
- Asthma Myths
- Useful Organizations

What Is Asthma?

A sthma is a chronic lung disease that can be controlled but not cured. The airways of people with asthma are supersensitive to things that don't bother other people with normal lungs. With asthma, the airways overreact to materials in the air (such as pollen, dust, pet dander, and smoke), to some respiratory infections, or even to cold air and exercise. These "triggers" cause the following problems:

- Inflammation, or swelling, of the walls of the airways
- Tightening or squeezing (*bronchospasm*) of the muscles surrounding the airways
- Excessive mucus production

This combination of swelling, squeezing, and extra mucus narrows, or obstructs, the airways and makes it difficult to inhale and exhale air.

Symptoms and Flares

The main symptoms of asthma are **shortness of breath, wheezing** (a high-pitched whistling sound with breathing), **coughing,** and **chest tightness.**

Many different patterns of symptoms exist. Symptoms usually come in new waves called **"flares,"** or attacks. Everyone with asthma has flares, but some individuals have more than others. Some people have no problems between flares, but many have symptoms every day. This is called "persistent" asthma, and its common cause is continuous exposure to triggers. For other people, symptoms may seem to go away for months or even years, but everyone with asthmatic lungs is at risk for new problems.

Asthma Triggers

There are five major groups of triggers:

1. **Infections,** such as colds and sinus infections; everyone with asthma has a problem with this trigger

2. **Allergies** to pollen (from trees, grass, weeds), molds, pet dander, dust mites, and cockroaches

3. **Irritants,** such as tobacco smoke, perfume, or chemical fumes from heaters

4. **Exercise**

5. **Cold air**

Treatment

Asthma is treated with two general categories of medicine:

1. Long-term **controller** medicines, usually taken on a daily basis to prevent airway inflammation, and

2. **Quick-relief** (or "rescue") medicines to treat symptoms as soon as they appear. (See chapter 5 for a review of both types of asthma medicines.)

The key to managing asthma is **keeping it under control** by avoiding triggers and using controller and quick relief medicines as prescribed.

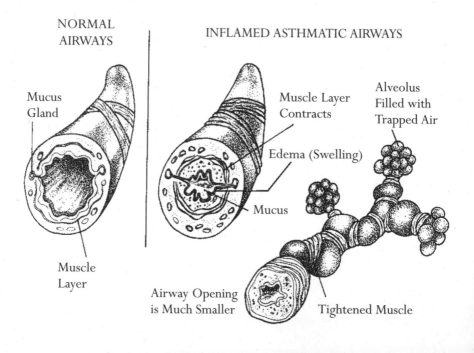

NORMAL AIRWAYS

INFLAMED ASTHMATIC AIRWAYS

Mucus Gland

Muscle Layer Contracts

Alveolus Filled with Trapped Air

Edema (Swelling)

Mucus

Muscle Layer

Airway Opening is Much Smaller

Tightened Muscle

A REVIEW OF THE
ALLERGY-ASTHMA CONNECTION

What are allergics?

Allergies are a very common problem that affect at least two out of every ten Americans. Allergies are a reaction of the body's immune system to substances that don't cause a reaction in people who don't have allergies. Your immune system, in effect, is responding to a false alarm. These substances trigger the immune system and the body to sneeze, wheeze, cough, and itch, depending on what part of your body has the reaction.

What is an allergen?

An allergen is any substance that leads to allergies by starting an immune response. Allergens are often common, usually harmless substances such as pollen, mold spores, animal dander, dust, foods, insect venoms, and some medicines. For more details about allergens, see chapter 3.

What causes the symptoms?

People with allergies have an allergic antibody called IgE (immunoglobulin E) in their bodies. IgE attaches or binds to the allergen and activates cells including "mast cells." After mast cells bind to the allergen and IgE, then the mast cells release chemicals called "mediators." One mediator—histamine—causes redness, swelling, and itching. The released mediators in the skin cause hives, in the nose sneezing, and in the lungs coughing and wheezing.

There is a strong connection between allergies and asthma. Most children with asthma also have allergies. A little less than half of people with allergic rhinitis (hay fever) have asthma symptoms, and half the people with atopic dermatitis (eczema) develop asthma. For many of them, the same allergen can trigger asthma, allergic rhinitis, and atopic dermatitis. In general, if allergic rhinitis is treated, asthma symptoms improve.

195

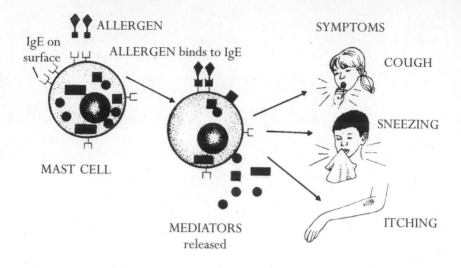

What are the common allergic diseases associated with asthma?

Symptoms of allergic rhinitis (hay fever) are nasal stuffiness, sneezing, nasal itching, clear runny nose, and itching of the roof of the mouth. One of the most common complications of allergic rhinitis is ear infection. As many as half of children over five years of age with chronic ear infections have confirmed allergic rhinitis.

Atopic dermatitis (eczema) is a chronic or recurrent inflammatory skin disease characterized by red lesions, scaling and dry flaking skin. In children, an allergy or irritant may aggravate it.

Food allergy is most commonly seen in very young children and is frequently outgrown. Food allergies are characterized by a broad range of allergic reactions including itching or swelling of lips or tongue; tightness of the throat with hoarseness; nausea and vomiting; diarrhea; occasionally chest tightness and wheezing; itching of the eyes; or even severe reaction like anaphylaxis. Food allergies very rarely cause asthma symptoms by themselves.

What is allergy testing?

An allergist can test your skin or sometimes your blood to determine if you have any allergies. Scratch or puncture tests are done on the surface of the skin. A tiny amount of allergen is scratched across or lightly pricked into the skin. If you have an allergy, swelling occurs only in the spots where the tiny amount of allergen to which you are allergic has been scratched onto your skin. For example, if you are allergic to dust mites but not to tree pollen, the spot where the dust mite allergen scratched your skin will swell and itch a bit, forming a small dime-size hive. The spot where the tree pollen allergen was scratched will not change.

Other types of testing include blood tests or intradermal (below the skin's surface) testing. The intradermal test is related to the scratch or puncture test, but it is slightly more sensitive. It involves injecting a tiny amount of allergen under the skin, usually on the upper arms. The diagnosis of allergies is not based only on skin testing. You can also have allergies based on symptoms even if all your skin tests are negative.

What are the treatment choices?

1. **Controlling the environment.** The first step is to identify allergens and then take steps to avoid or control them as much as possible. Simple measures in your home can reduce your exposure to indoor allergens. Avoiding outdoor allergens is more difficult, as pollens can travel hundreds of miles. (More details on control and avoidance of allergens are discussed in chapter 10.)

2. **Medicines.** Taking medicines, either prescribed or over-the-counter, that counteract or block the reaction and reduce or eliminate the symptoms. Numerous medicines are available and relief is possible for many people.

3. **Allergy vaccination or "allergy shots."** Allergy injection therapy works like an immunization shot against the allergens that you are allergic to. Although this is extremely helpful for some people, this form of therapy is usually reserved for people with severe allergies or people who have tried different treatments that have not worked.

FREQUENTLY ASKED QUESTIONS ABOUT ASTHMA

Following are answers to some of the questions that parents most often ask about their child's asthma:

Q. Can asthma be cured?

A. No, asthma cannot be cured. Some children can "outgrow" wheezing and coughing; they may not have asthma to begin with. Asthma is a chronic disease that can be controlled and managed. Although asthma concerns parents most when they see their child experiencing symptoms or having problems breathing, the child still has some degree of airway inflammation even when well. If a child is not experiencing symptoms, it is not because the asthma has gone away but because it is under control.

Q. Can you catch asthma from someone?

A. No, asthma is not an infectious or contagious disease.

Q. Are some people more likely to have asthma than others?

A. Asthma can affect anyone, young or old, male or female, people of all races and ethnic backgrounds. When one or both parents have asthma, a child has a greater chance of also having the lung disease. But many children develop asthma without any family history of the disease.

Q. I have not heard anything good about steroids. Why are steroids used to treat asthma, especially in children, if they are so "dangerous"? Aren't all steroids the same? What about the steroids that athletes take?

A. There are different types of steroids. One important fact to consider is that the human body manufactures steroids, and we can't live without them. Steroids taken and abused by athletes to grow bigger and stronger are *not* the same as steroids used to treat asthma. Most of the bad side effects of steroids that people hear about—puffy, swollen face (especially the cheeks), high blood pressure, behavior changes, acne, skin thinning, bruising, stomach upset/ulcer, osteoporosis, cataracts, glaucoma, reduced ability to fight infections, and growth suppression come from long-term treatment (not a three-to five-day course or burst) with prednisone taken by mouth, not inhaled steroids.

Prednisone is used to treat children with asthma for a short burst when they have an asthma flare or longer in some cases of severe asthma. If a child takes prednisone for a few days and develops side effects, the side effects usually resolve after finishing it. Prednisone is dosed in milligrams per kilogram of a child's body weight. Inhaled steroids are dosed in micrograms (it takes 1,000 micrograms to equal 1 milligram). In other words, the dose of inhaled steroids is very small. It is delivered directly to the lungs, where it is needed. It does not go through the whole body. Through research, we know that inhaled steroids are the best medicine we have to treat asthma.

Q. Can someone die from asthma?

A. Yes, asthma can be fatal, but fortunately this is rare. When asthma is the cause of death, it is usually because patients didn't take their medicines properly (when and how they were supposed to), or they didn't get help in time because they didn't take their symptoms seriously.

Q. It seems like more and more children are being diagnosed with asthma. Why is that happening?

A. Asthma is the most common chronic disease of childhood, and the number one reason that children miss school, go to emergency rooms, and are admitted to hospitals. About five million American children are estimated to have asthma, and the number continues to rise worldwide. We don't know why this is happening even though many asthma experts are doing research to try to find out. Some of the reasons for the increase may be that asthma is better recognized and diagnosed than in the past; increased air pollution; homes with less ventilation, more moisture, more indoor pets, and children spending more time indoors.

Q. My child always seems to have a cold and now has been diagnosed with asthma. How do I know the difference between a cold and asthma?

A. A cold is an upper respiratory tract infection caused by a virus. Colds are a common asthma trigger; in fact they are the most common trigger in babies and toddlers. Usually when a youngster gets a cold, the cold will last a week or less. When a child with uncontrolled asthma catches a cold, the cold triggers the asthma. So although the cold itself is gone in a few days or a week, the child's cold seems to go on and on because of asthma symptoms, such as coughing and wheezing. In uncontrolled asthma, this coughing and wheezing can last for weeks. Before you know it (especially in the winter), the child gets another cold—although it seems like the last one never went away. All of us catch colds, so make sure when your child gets a cold that you follow his or her action plan to treat symptoms and keep them under control.

Q. What is the best way to give inhaled asthma medicine?

A. There is no one-size-fits-all answer. Some children do well when given medicine by nebulizer machine and others by an inhaler with a spacer. There are pros and cons about each. Whichever device is prescribed, it must be used correctly to be effective. For example, if you use a nebulizer, it should be used with a face mask or mouthpiece; don't just blow the mist into the child's face. Research has shown that metered dose inhalers work well for infants if used with a spacer and face mask.

Q. Can my child become addicted to asthma medicine?

A. No, asthma medicines are not addictive.

Q. How can I tell when to replace my child's equipment: air compressor, filter, nebulizer tubing with mouthpiece or face mask?

A. When you get new equipment, keep the instruction booklet. If your child uses a nebulizer and air compressor, make sure you keep the phone number of the company that supplied the equipment. The manufacturers of any piece of equipment will include information about how long it should last. To replace equipment, you will need a prescription. In order for the equipment to be covered by insurance, make sure that you order from a pharmacy or equipment company that has a contract with your insurance provider.

You need to know if your child's nebulizer tubing and medicine cup are disposable or reusable and how long you can use them. Follow the instructions to clean and disinfect the nebulizer. And remember: if you don't follow the manufacturer's instruction regarding maintenance and replacement of parts, it will affect the performance of the machine and the treatment your child receives.

A spacer should last at least one year and maybe longer if it is cleaned properly, is not cracked or otherwise damaged, and the one-way valve remains intact. All spacers come with instructions about how to clean them. Not cleaning them properly will affect their performance.

Q. When should my child stop playing or come out of gym or a game because of asthma symptoms?

A. There should be no restrictions on children's ability to play, take gym class, or compete in sports just because they have asthma. If your child has been instructed to take medicine before physical activity, however, make sure that he or she does so every time. Some parents hesitate to give medicine before exercise or sports because their child seems fine or is active and doesn't develop symptoms.

Remember: you are giving the medicine to *prevent* symptoms and start your child off at her best, so she can participate actively with other children. Check with your nurse practitioner or doctor first, but in general, if a child experiences symptoms while playing, she should stop and take her quick-relief medicine. If she feels better and the medicine relieves the symptoms, she should be able to resume the activity. If the symptoms return, she should stop playing and you should follow the instructions in her action plan.

Q. My child only has occasional seasonal symptoms and seems fine most of the time, so why does he need to take medicine every day?

A. Many parents feel this way, but don't forget that asthma is a chronic disease. It's ongoing—it's there every day, even when the child feels fine and has no symptoms. One way to decide whether a child needs medicine daily is to go by the guidelines recommended by the

National Institutes of Health. These guidelines were written by a group of experts who reviewed research about asthma and made treatment recommendations. The guidelines recommend that if a child has symptoms more than twice a week and/or three or more flares within a year, then the child should be given daily controller medicine and monitored carefully. Remember, guidelines are recommendations and each child should be viewed as an individual, so if you have questions about this, talk to your child's nurse practitioner or pediatrician.

Q. How do I know when to refill my child's inhalers? It seems like they are all different.

A. Yes, different medicines are produced by different manufacturers. You just need to be familiar with your own child's medicines. The newer, dry powder inhalers have a dose counter or indicator to let you know when they need to be refilled.

The best way to know when other inhalers are running out is to count puffs. For example, Flovent inhalers come with 120 "actuations," or puffs of medicine, because the recommended dose is two puffs twice a day, which equals four puffs a day total. If there are 120 puffs in the canister and you divide 120 by 4, the inhaler will last thirty days. After thirty days you may still feel liquid in the canister and you may see liquid spray out, but the medicine is gone and the liquid is the leftover propellant and preservative—so replace it.

Most albuterol inhalers come with 200 puffs of medicine or 100 (two-puff) doses. The usual dose of albuterol is two puffs as needed. If a child's asthma is under control, he should only be using albuterol before exercise and on an as-needed basis twice a week or less often. The best way to know when your child's albuterol is running out is to count puffs. For example, if a child takes a two-puff dose of albuterol once a week before gym class, another two-puff dose once a week before soccer, and two puffs twice a week for symptoms, that equals four (two-puff) doses for a total of eight puffs a week, and the albuterol inhaler should last twenty-five weeks (six months).

If you are unsure about how best to keep track of when to refill your child's inhalers, talk to your pharmacist, who can instruct you about when to get refills.

Q. Why does my child seem to have more asthma symptoms at night? I would have expected he'd have more coughing and wheezing when he's running around during the daytime.

A. The body's protective mechanisms against airway inflammation decrease between midnight and early morning because blood levels of cortisol and epinephrine, which are naturally occurring hormones, decrease at night—thereby allowing inflammation to increase. If your child has nighttime cough, wheezing, or shortness of breath, talk with your doctor or nurse practitioner about the use of anti-inflammatory corticosteroids if your child isn't already using them; if your child does take them as a controller medicine, your doctor may recommend an increased dose when necessary.

Q. I'm trying to quit smoking, but it's difficult. I know it's not good for my child to be around cigarette smoke, so I go outside to smoke, but he still seems to cough and breathe shallowly when he's around me.

A. A lot of parents think they're not exposing their children to second-hand smoke if they only smoke outdoors, but the smoke still sticks to your hair, clothing, and skin. So if you cuddle up with your child as you're reading him a bedtime story, don't be surprised if the smoke particles trigger asthma symptoms.

Keep trying to quit smoking for the sake of your own health as well as your child's, but if you really can't quit, at least try to wear a "smoking jacket" when you go outside to smoke and put it away when you come back indoors. Wash your hands and face after smoking, especially if you're going to be in close contact with your child. And ask other people not to smoke inside your home or around your child.

Q. We've had some scary episodes with my child's asthma in the past, but now it's been under good control for months. The nurse is always urging me to bring my child back for a checkup, though. I'm really busy with work. Are follow-up appointments really that important?

A. Yes, they are. When a child hasn't had a flare for a while, it's easy to assume everything is okay. But follow-up visits are important because asthma never really goes away. These appointments help you continue to learn about your child's pattern of asthma symptoms and how they might be changing. They also can determine whether lung function tests are remaining stable or improving or whether daily controller medicines might need adjusting to the lowest effective doses.

At follow-up visits, your doctor or nurse practitioner can discuss any side effects and make sure that the medicines are being taken properly, including spacer use. They can answer any questions or concerns you might have and identify any problems you may have with getting the care you need: insurance coverage, access to appointments, ability to get medicines, organizing the medicine schedule. So it's important to keep those follow-up appointments as part of your ongoing effort to keep your child healthy.

A REVIEW OF
ASTHMA MEDICINES

Two General Types of Asthma Medicine

1. **Controller** (or anti-inflammatory) medicines reduce the swelling, squeezing, and extra mucus in the airways. They are long-term treatments taken to **prevent** and control symptoms. When first started, these medicines usually take time to work, sometimes weeks. They will do two things:

- **Prevent everyday problems** during the times between flares.
- **Reduce flares**, both the number and severity.

Do not stop the daily anti-inflammatory medicines until your doctor recommends it. If you stop these medicines after you gain control, inflammation might return, along with symptoms and more flares.

Examples of controller medicines include **inhaled steroids** (e.g., Flovent and Pulmicort). There are also **nonsteroid** anti-inflammatory medicines, including "leukotriene modifiers" (Singulair and Accolate) and another group that includes Intal (cromolyn) and Tilade.

Another type of medicine, called **"long-acting bronchodilators,"** help control asthma symptoms because they stay active over time. But these medicines do not act fast enough for quick relief, so they are **not used in treatment of new flares**. Long-acting bronchodilators are not anti-inflammatory medicines when given by themselves, but they can help inhaled steroids to work when both are prescribed together.

2. **Quick-relief medicines** work very differently. They are **short-acting** bronchodilators that open the airways by relaxing the muscles that surround them. These bronchodilators are used for quick relief of asthma symptoms. They come in an inhaler or nebulizer form. Examples include Proventil and Ventolin (or albuterol), and the newer drug Xopenex (levalbuterol). Sometimes quick-relief medicines are also called "rescue" or "reliever" medicines.

Oral steroid anti-inflammatories, such as Liquid Pred, Deltasone (prednisone), prednisolone, or methylprednisolone, are used if an asthma flare is not brought under control by increased use of inhaled corticosteroids or quick-relief medicines, and in cases of severe asthma that are very difficult to control over time.

Your child's pediatrician, nurse practitioner, or asthma specialist will discuss how the medicines work, when to use them, what to expect, and how to recognize any side effects. You will need to learn about them before becoming comfortable and knowledgeable enough to use them safely and effectively.

Remember: The Goals of Treatment

- Minimal symptoms or problems between flares. The goal is none!
- No limits in physical activities, including participation in exercise and sports.
- Fewer flares and easier control of new flares.
- Sleeping through the night.
- Fewer absences from school and work.
- The ability to self-manage asthma to the greatest extent possible, for parent and child.
- No side effects from asthma medicines.

ASTHMA MEDICINES

The following table lists various asthma medicines by type, generic and brand names, delivery method, and possible side effects.

Controller Medicines (long-term)

Type	Generic Name	Brand Name	Method/ Device	Possible Side Effects
Anti-inflammatory inhaled steroids	Fluticasone	Flovent	Inhaler	Oral thrush, (yeast infection), dry cough (rare)
	Beclomethasone	Vanceril, Beclovent, Qvar	Inhaler	
	Triamcinolone	Azmacort	Inhaler	
	Flunisolide	AeroBid	Inhaler	
	Budesonide	Pulmicort Turbuhaler	Nebulizer Inhaler	
Anti-inflammatory leukotriene modifiers	Montelukast	Singulair	Pill	Nausea (rare), fever
	Zafirlukast	Accolate	Pill	
Anti-inflammatory nonsteroids	Cromolyn	Intal	Inhaler or nebulizer	Dry cough (rare)
	Nedocromil	Tilade		
Long-acting bronchodilator	Salmeterol	Serevent	Inhaler or Diskus	Shakiness, nervousness, fast heartbeat
Bronchodilator	Theophylline	Slo-bid, Theo-24, Slo-phylline	Capsules or intravenous	Nausea, stomachache, fast heartbeat
Combined medicines (steroid, anti-inflammatory and long-acting bronchodilator)	Salmeterol, Fluticasone	Advair	Diskus	Dry mouth, thrush, jitteriness

Quick-Relief Medicines

Type	Generic Name	Brand Name	Method/ Device	Side Effects
Bronchodilator	Albuterol	Proventil, Ventolin	Inhaler or nebulizer	Fast heartbeat, shakiness, nervousness, stomachache
	Levalbuterol	Xopenex	Nebulizer	
Anti-inflammatory oral steroids	Prednisone	Liquid Pred, Deltasone	Liquid or pills	Increased appetite, increased weight, jitteriness, mood changes; all reversible
	Prednisolone	Prelone, Pediapred, Orapred	Liquid	
	Methylprednisolone	Medrol	Pill	
	Dexamethasone	Decadron and others	Pill or liquid	

Medicines are marketed under many names. A "generic" name can refer to the chemical name of a medicine that is available under several different brand names. Some medicines, whose patents have expired, are marketed under other generic names. Ask your physician or pharmacist for clarification about names of your child's medicines.

A GUIDE TO USING SPACERS

Medicine to treat asthma can be delivered in several ways—inhaled or in pill or liquid form. The one you're probably most familiar with is the metered dose inhaler (MDI) with a spacer (also called a "holding chamber") attached as a delivery device.

Q. Who should use a spacer?

A. All children who take asthma medicine with MDIs should use spacers. They come with face masks for babies and toddlers or a mouthpiece for older children.

Q. Why does a child need a spacer?

A. A spacer helps the medicine get deep into the lungs where it needs to go to work on swollen, squeezed, and inflamed airways. MDIs deliver medicine in an aerosol spray that comes out very fast. The attached spacer holds the spray so a child can inhale it slowly and get it deep down into the lungs. With a spacer, less medicine stays in the mouth and throat.

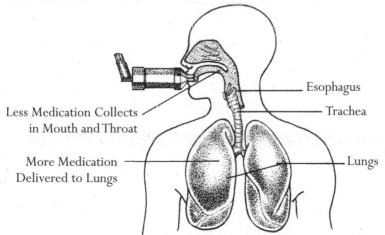

Less Medication Collects in Mouth and Throat

More Medication Delivered to Lungs

Esophagus

Trachea

Lungs

Q. How do I get a spacer?

A. Ask your child's nurse practitioner or doctor for a prescription. Most pharmacies carry spacers. Some health insurance plans cover the cost of spacers, and others don't. Call your health care plan provider to find out if spacers are covered and where to get them.

Q. How should a spacer be cleaned?

A. Instructions for cleaning should be enclosed in the box with the spacer. Don't put a spacer in the dishwasher. Most spacers should be washed once a week with dishwashing soap, rinsed well, and allowed to air-dry.

Q. How can a parent be sure a child is using a spacer the right way?

A. At your next medical appointment, ask your child's doctor or nurse to demonstrate the correct technique *and* give you written instructions to take home. At each visit, take your spacer and inhaler along and ask the doctor or nurse to watch your child demonstrate how he uses his MDI/spacer. If he's using it incorrectly, he can be reinstructed; this will help you supervise its proper use at home.

How to Use a Metered Dose Inhaler (MDI) with a Spacer

1. Get your MDI and spacer and check your asthma management plan for instructions about when to take medcine. Is the MDI running low? Call for refills before running out.

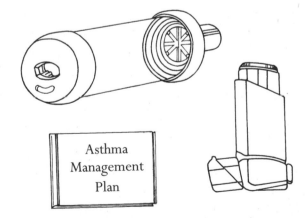

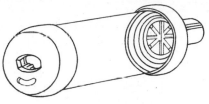

2. Check the spacer:
   Is it clean, cracked,
   or broken? Make
   sure it's empty and
   no foreign objects
   are inside.

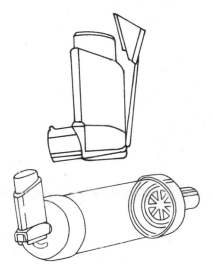

3. Remove the caps
   from both the
   MDI and the
   spacer. Put the
   MDI in the soft
   rubber ring of the
   spacer. Shake the
   MDI and spacer
   four or five times.

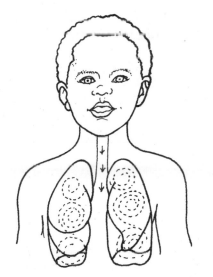

4. Take one breath in
   and one breath out.

5. Place the spacer
   mouth piece in
   your mouth with
   the MDI canister
   pointing upward.

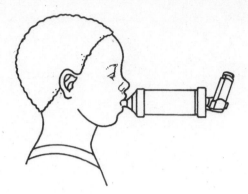

6. Push the MDI
   down so one
   puff of medi-
   cine is sprayed
   into the spacer.

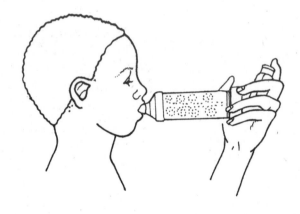

7. Take one *slow,*
   deep breath in.
   (If you hear a
   whistle, you are
   inhaling too fast.)
   Hold the breath
   for ten seconds.

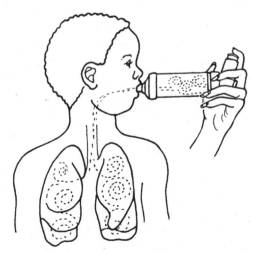

8. If two puffs of medicine have been prescribed, repeat steps 3 through 7.

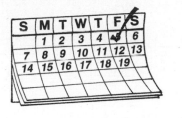

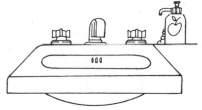

9. Keep the spacer clean. Most spacers should be washed once a week with dishwashing soap, rinsed, and air dried. Check the manufacturer's directions for more information.

How to Use a Metered Dose Inhaler (MDI) with a Spacer and Face Mask

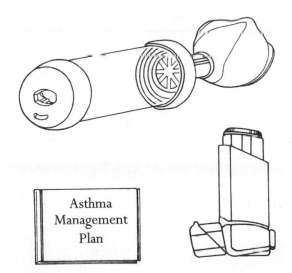

1. Get your child's MDI and spacer with attached face mask. Check your child's asthma management plan for instructions about when to give medicine. Is the MDI running low? Call for refills before running out.

Asthma Management Plan

2. Check the spacer. Is it clean, cracked, or broken? Make sure it is empty and no foreign objects are inside.

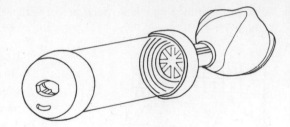

3. Remove the cap from the MDI; put the MDI canister in the rubber ring at the open end of the spacer with the canister pointing upward.

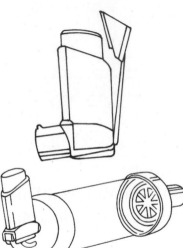

4. Sit your child on your lap; shake the MDI/spacer/face mask four or five times.

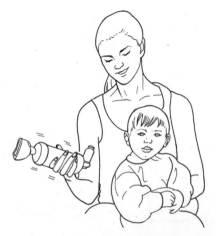

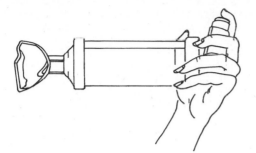

5. Push down on the MDI so one puff of medicine is sprayed into the spacer.

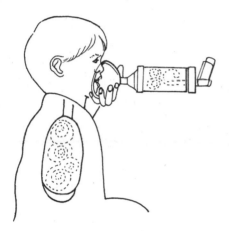

6. Immediately place the mask gently over your child's face and make sure that it is sealed over his mouth and nose. Be certain that there is a good seal. Don't worry—your child can breathe in and out comfortably with the mask sealed in place.

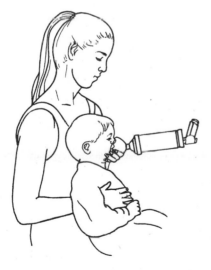

7. Keep the mask in place by anchoring your hand under your child's chin until he breathes in and out *six times*. You'll know that he has gotten the medicine and taken six breaths by watching his chest move in and out or by placing your hand on his belly and feeling it go up and down six times.

8. If two puffs of medicine have been prescribed, repeat steps 4 through 7. You'll know your child has gotten the medicine and taken six breaths by watching his chest move in and out or by placing your hand on his belly and feeling it go up and down six times.

9. Keep the spacer clean. Most spacers should be washed once a week with dishwashing soap, rinsed, and air dried. Check the manufacturer's directions for additional information.

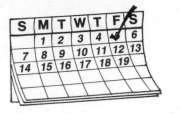

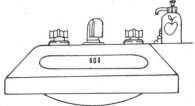

A Guide to Using
a Peak Flow Meter

A peak flow meter measures how well air moves in and out of the lungs. It is particularly useful because it acts as an "early warning system" that can detect any squeezing in the airways hours or even days before symptoms of asthma actually appear.

If you measure your child's peak flow regularly—even when your child feels fine—you can determine whether her asthma is well controlled or if control is slipping. Regular use of a peak flow meter won't prevent an asthma flare, but it can give a warning of worsening symptoms.

The peak flow meter can also be used to help you and your doctor or nurse practitioner:

- Identify factors that can trigger your asthma symptoms
- Talk about your asthma with more knowledge
- Decide how well your treatment plan is working
- Decide when to add or stop medicine
- Decide when to seek emergency care

Children five years of age and older who have moderate to severe asthma should check their peak flow meters regularly. Ask your child's doctor or nurse to show you how to use a peak flow meter. They will also help you develop an asthma management plan to keep your child's asthma under control and treat symptoms when they arise. The plan will include your child's "personal best" peak flow reading, described on the next page.

How to Use a Peak Flow Meter

1. Get your peak
   flow meter and
   peak flow record.

Peak Flow Record

2. Place the indicator at 0
   or the bottom of the
   numbered scale.

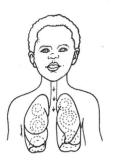

0

3. Stand up. Take a
   deep breath.

4. Put the meter in your
   mouth and close your
   lips around the mouth-
   piece. Keep your
   tongue on the bottom
   of your mouth, not over
   the hole in the mouth-
   piece. Blow out as hard
   and fast as you can!

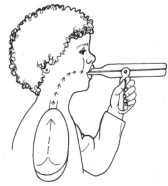

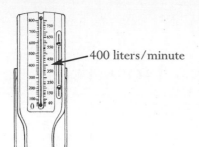

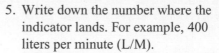 400 liters/minute

5. Write down the number where the indicator lands. For example, 400 liters per minute (L/M).

6. Repeat steps 1 through 6 two more times.

7. Write down your highest peak flow reading in your peak flow record.

  Trial 1: _____ L/M
  Trial 2: _____ L/M
  Trial 3: _____ L/M

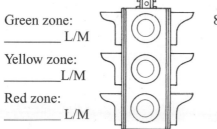

Green zone:
_____ L/M

Yellow zone:
_____L/M

Red zone:
_____ L/M

8. Check what zone your peak flow reading is in.

Personal best: _____ L/M.

You and your child's doctor should decide what your child's "personal best" peak flow reading is.

9. Check your child's asthma management plan to see if you need to make any medicine adjustments based on your child's peak flow reading.

  Green zone: Take long-term control medicines
  Yellow zone: Start action plan
  Red zone: Continue action plan and call or go to the ER

Your child's "personal best" peak flow number is the highest reading your child can reach over a two-week period when her asthma is under good control. Good control means that your child feels good and has no asthma symptoms.

Remember:

The green zone is 80 to 100 percent of your child's personal best peak flow reading.

The yellow zone is 50 to 80 percent of your child's personal best peak flow reading.

The red zone is less than 50 percent of your child's personal best peak flow reading.

Discuss these readings with your child's doctor.

THE CHILDREN'S HOSPITAL
OF PHILADELPHIA'S
ASTHMA MANAGEMENT PLAN

Child's name _____

Date _____

Everyday medicines (Green Zone—peak flow 80 to 100 percent of personal best: _____ – _____)

Give these *controller (anti-inflammatory)* medicines every day, to prevent problems, even when your child is well!

Medicine/How much to give?/How often?

❏ Flovent inhaler: _____ mcg with a spacer _____ puffs _____ times a day

❏ Pulmicort Turbuhaler: _____ puffs _____ times a day

❏ Pulmicort Respules: _____ mg by nebulizer _____ vials _____ times a day

❏ Advair Diskus: _____ puffs _____ times a day

❏ Singulair tablet: _____ mg one tablet once a day

❏ Serevent inhaler: _____ mcg with a spacer _____ puffs _____ times a day

❏ Other: _____ _____ _____ times a day

Remember to rinse your mouth out after taking inhaled medicines!

If you have trouble breathing during exercise or sports, use

❏ Albuterol inhaler with a spacer: _____ puffs 15–30 minutes before exercise

❏ _____ _____ puffs 15–30 minutes before exercise

220

When symptoms start

For cough, wheezing, shortness of breath, or chest tightness use a *quick-relief (bronchodilator)* medicine:

❏ Albuterol inhaler with a spacer: _____ puffs up to every 4 hours as needed

❏ _____ by nebulizer, one premixed vial up to every 4 hours as needed

❏ Albuterol: _____ ml in _____ by nebulizer, one dose up to every 4 hours as needed

If quick-relief medicine is used more than once a day, a flare may be starting!

Action plan for flares (Yellow Zone—peak flow reading between 50 and 80 percent of personal best: _____ – _____)

1. Continue to use *quick-relief (bronchodilator)* medicines

❏ Albuterol inhaler with a spacer _____ puffs up to every 4 hours as needed

❏ _____ by nebulizer, one pre-mixed vial up to every 4 hours as needed

❏ Albuterol: _____ ml in _____ by nebulizer, one dose up to every 4 hours as needed

AND

2. Give extra *controller (anti-inflammatory)* medicine for _____ days

❏ Flovent MDI _____ with a spacer _____ puffs _____ times a day

❏ Pulmicort Turbuhaler: _____ puffs _____ times a day

❏ Pulmicort Respules: _____ mg by nebulizer, _____ vials _____ times a day

❏ Advair Diskus: _____ _____ puffs _____ times a day

❏ Prednisone: _____ mg _____ times a day

3. Continue these everyday *controller (anti-inflammatory)* medicines:

_____

Call your doctor's office if the symptoms don't improve in two days or if the flare lasts longer than _____ days.

Danger

**Red Zone—if peak flow is lower than 50 percent of your personal best
(_____), or if asthma *symptoms are getting worse*, breathing is hard
and fast, you cannot talk, or feel that the medicine is not helping, use:**

❏ Albuterol _____ puffs by spacer *or* one vial by nebulizer *and*
  call _____

**If you cannot reach anyone, call 911
or go to the nearest emergency room!**

ELIMINATING ASTHMA TRIGGERS

The following list can help families decrease or eliminate allergens and irritants that trigger asthma symptoms. You may want to make copies of this list, take a pencil, and occasionally walk through your home to check for any trigger suspects.

In the Child's Bedroom

- Remove carpets if possible; damp-mop hardwood or linoleum floors often.
- If rugs can't be removed, use a vacuum with a good filter or double-thick bags; don't vacuum while the child is in the room.
- Replace draperies, slats, or blinds with wipeable pull-down window shades to reduce dust.
- Wipe down baseboards, molding, windowsills, shelves, and other surfaces with a damp cloth to catch dust.
- Remove dust collectors (stuffed toys, books, magazines, and clutter), or store them—especially each night—in a closed container, cupboard, or closet.
- In hot weather, use an air conditioner rather than a fan in an open window.
- Encase mattresses and pillows in plastic or special "vapo-permeable" fine-weave fabrics; use pillows made of synthetic materials, not feather pillows. Encase box springs in vinyl or plastic.
- Keep pets out of the child's bedroom at all times, whether the child is present or not.
- Wash all sheets, pillowcases, blankets, comforters, and mattress pads in hot water (130°F) every week or ten days. (Only hot water kills dust mites.)

In the Kitchens and Bathrooms

- Air out and frequently clean damp areas with chlorine bleach to eliminate mold and mildew.

- Clean tile and grout often.
- Clean under sinks and behind toilets regularly.
- Fix any dripping faucets or leaks so water doesn't collect.
- Seal cracks and remove any source of standing water (such as a refrigerator drip pan).
- Store food in sealed containers.
- Wash dishes daily; don't leave them in the sink.
- Put trash outside nightly or daily.
- Use traps or pesticides to kill cockroaches or call an exterminator; keep areas dry because dampness attracts cockroaches.

In Other Living Areas
- Select vinyl, leather, plastic, or wood furniture instead of upholstered furniture where possible, especially in rooms where children are most likely to sit. Don't let your child with asthma lie down or sleep on an upholstered sofa, for example. Avoid throw pillows.
- Remove carpets, particularly in areas where children spend a lot of time—family room, den. If that's not possible, vacuum weekly with a machine that has a good filter, and don't vacuum while the child is in the room.
- Select curtains or drapes made of synthetic rather than natural fibers, or use shades or window blinds that can be wiped or washed regularly.
- Dust with a damp cloth to avoid stirring up dust.
- Check houseplants and dried floral arrangements for dust and mold.
- Try to reduce humidity throughout the home with air-conditioning or a dehumidifier.

In the Basement
- Eliminate dampness or dripping water to reduce mold; seal cracks.
- Don't use carpeting in usually damp areas or on concrete-slab basement floors.
- Consider using a dehumidifier (with the humidity level set between 25 and 50 percent) in damp basements; clean and empty dehumidifier regularly.
- Don't let a child with asthma sleep in a basement room.

Heating, Cooling, and Filtering Systems

- Use an air conditioner if possible to keep pollen from entering your home and to keep indoor humidity low.
- Clean or replace air conditioner and furnace filters routinely.
- If you use an air filter, such as a portable HEPA (high-energy particulate air) filter, place it only on a bare, clean floor—not on a carpet.

Pets

Find a new home for your cat, dog, bird, or pet rodent. Consider replacing it with a type of pet that doesn't cause allergies, such as tropical fish, reptiles, hermit crabs. But if you absolutely cannot part with your furry or feathered friend:

- Keep it outdoors as much as possible.
- *Never* let the pet in the bedroom of a child with asthma, even if the child isn't in the room at the time.
- If the pet is allowed indoors, confine it to a room with a bare—not carpeted—floor. Keep it off sofas and beds.
- Wash the pet weekly in warm water.

Special Irritants around the Home

Avoid strong odors and other irritants such as:

- Tobacco smoke
- Woodsmoke
- Strong perfumes, talcum powder, hair spray, cleaning products
- Paint fumes
- Strong cooking odors, particularly from frying foods

A School Management Plan

The following model of a School Management Plan can be duplicated, filled out, and signed by parent/guardian and your child's physician. The completed form should be given to your child's teacher, school nurse, coach, day care or after-school supervisor, camp counselor, and anyone else who has regular contact with and responsibility for your child with asthma.

```
┌─ ─ ─ ─ ─ ─ ─ ─ ─┐
|                 |
|                 |
|                 |
|   ID photo      |
|                 |
|                 |
|                 |
└─ ─ ─ ─ ─ ─ ─ ─ ─┘
```

Asthma School Management Plan for _____

Grade: _____   Age: _____

Teacher: _____   Room: _____

Parent/   Parent/
  guardian: _____   guardian: _____

Home phone: _____   Home phone: _____

Work/cell phone: _____   Work/cell phone: _____

Emergency Contacts

1. Name: _____   Phone: _____
   Relationship: _____

2. Name: _____   Phone: _____
   Relationship: _____

Physician student
  sees for asthma: _____   Phone: _____

Other physician: _____   Phone: _____

Daily Asthma Management Plan

Identify things that may trigger asthma symptoms (wheezing, coughing, shortness of breath, chest tightness). Check each that applies to this student:

226

❏ Respiratory infections
❏ Exercise
❏ Animals
❏ Pollens
❏ Molds

❏ Strong odors or fumes
❏ Carpets in the room
❏ Chalk dust
❏ Other _____

Peak Flow Monitoring
Personal best peak flow number _____
Monitoring times: _____ _____ _____

Daily Medication Plan

Name of Medicine	Amount	When to Use
1. _____	_____	_____
2. _____	_____	_____
3. _____	_____	_____

Comments/special instructions:

_____

_____

_____

_____

Emergency Plan
Emergency treatment is necessary when the student has symptoms such as _____ or has a peak flow meter reading below _____.

Take these steps during an asthma flare or attack:
1. Give medicines as listed in the next section.
2. Have the student return to classroom if _____
3. Contact parent if _____
4. **Seek emergency medical care if the student has any of the following:**
   - No improvement 15 to 20 minutes after initial treatment with medicine and a relative cannot be reached
   - Peak flow of _____

- Hard time breathing (any of the scenarios below):
  Chest and neck pulled in with breathing
  Child is hunched over
  Child is struggling to breathe
- Trouble walking or talking
- Stops playing and can't start activity again
- Lips or fingernails are gray or blue

Emergency Asthma Medicines

	Name of Medicine	Amount	When to Use
1.	_____	_____	_____
2.	_____	_____	_____
3.	_____	_____	_____
4.	_____	_____	_____

Comments/special instructions:

_____

_____

_____

For Inhaled Medicines

I have instructed _____ in the proper way to use his/her medicines. It is my professional opinion that _____ should be allowed to carry and use these medicines by him/herself.

OR

It is my professional opinion that _____ should not carry his/her inhaled medicines by him/herself.

Physician's signature: _____ Date: _____

Parent's signature: _____ Date: _____

HOW ASTHMA-FRIENDLY IS YOUR
SCHOOL OR DAY CARE CENTER?

Parents do their best to keep their children healthy, but children also need support outside the home to keep their asthma under control and to participate fully in school and day care activities. The following list of questions can help parents work with school and day care staff to raise awareness of asthma control and assure a healthy, asthma-friendly environment.

- Is your school free of tobacco smoke all the time, even during school-sponsored events?

- Does your school maintain good indoor air quality? Does it reduce or eliminate allergens and irritants that bother children with asthma?

- Does the school building have cockroaches? Mold? Dust mites (often found in carpets, upholstery, stuffed toys)? Is chalk dust a problem? Are there pets in the classroom? Strong odors or fumes from art supplies, cleaning chemicals, paint?

- Is a school nurse present in school all day, every day? If not, is one regularly available to monitor children's management plans and medicines, especially when physical education and field trips are involved?

- Can children take medicine at school as recommended by their doctors and parents?

- Are children allowed to carry their medicines with them?

- Does your school have a written emergency plan for taking care of a child who might have a severe asthma flare? Is it clear what to do? Who and when to call?

- Does someone teach the staff about asthma, management plans, and medicines? Does someone also teach other children about asthma and how to get help for a classmate who needs it?

- Do children have good options for fully, safely participating in recess and physical education? Do they have access to their medicines before exercising? Can they choose a modified or alternative activity when medically necessary?

FAMOUS PEOPLE WITH ASTHMA

Four U.S. presidents, various rock stars, Academy Award winners, Olympic gold medalists, Hall of Fame baseball players, Nobel Prize winners, and many other famous people are known to have asthma. They include:

Leaders in Science and Politics

Beruj Benacerraf, immunologist, Nobel Prize winner

Bill Clinton (has severe allergies), 42nd president of the United States

Calvin Coolidge, 30th president of the United States

Elias James Corey, Nobel Prize winner— Chemistry

Ernesto (Che) Guevara, Argentine-born freedom fighter

Oliver Wendell Holmes, physician, inventor, artist, teacher

Rev. Jesse Jackson, African American political leader

John Paul Jones, American Revolutionary War hero, father of the U.S. Navy

John F. Kennedy, 35th president of the United States

John Locke, British physician, philosopher

Walter F. Mondale, 42nd vice president of the United States

Peter the Great, Russian czar

Marcel Proust, 19th-century philosopher and writer

Theodore Roosevelt, 26th president of the United States

William Tecumseh Sherman, general in the Civil War's Union Army

Barbara Smith, writer, critic, publisher, activist

Martin Van Buren, 8th president of the United States

Daniel Webster, statesman and lawyer

King William III, King of England, Scotland

Woodrow Wilson, 28th president of the United States

The Arts

Jason Alexander, actor, director, singer, dancer

Steve Allen, comedian, musician, TV personality

Ludwig von Beethoven, German composer

Leonard Bernstein, composer, conductor, and pianist

Judy Collins, singer, pianist, author

Alice Cooper, rock musician, performer

Dani,
Sesame Street muppet

Jonathon Davis,
singer (Korn)

Charles Dickens,
British novelist

DMX, hip-hop artist

Morgan Fairchild,
actress

Kenny G,
saxophonist,
composer

Bob Hope,
comedian and film
actor

Billy Joel,
rock musician,
performer

Ricki Lake,
talk show host

Liza Minnelli,
actress, singer

Joseph Pulitzer,
publisher and
philanthropist

Christopher Reeve,
actor

Martin Scorsese,
film director

Paul Sorvino,
actor, tenor

Sharon Stone,
actress

Elizabeth Taylor,
actress

Dylan Thomas, Welsh
poet, playwright

John Updike, writer

Antonio Vivaldi,
Italian musician
and priest

Orson Welles, actor and
director

Athletes

Jerome "The Bus"
Bettis, NFL Pro Ball
running back

Bruce Davidson,
Olympic athlete
(equestrian)

Tom Dolan, Olympic
swimmer (gold
medalist)

Kurt Grote, Olympic
swimmer
(gold medalist)

Nancy Hogshead,
Olympic swimmer
(gold medalist)

Juwan Howard,
basketball player

Jim (Catfish) Hunter,
Hall of Fame baseball
player

Jackie Joyner-Kersee,
Olympic track and field
(gold medalist)

Bill Koch, Olympic
medalist in skiing

Greg Louganis,
olympic diver (gold
medalist)

Debbie Meyer,
Olympic swimmer
(triple gold medalist)

Art Monk, Hall of
Fame football player

George Murray,
wheelchair marathon
champion

Rob Muzzio, Olympic
athlete (decathlon)

Dennis Rodman,
basketball player

Emmitt Smith, NFL
Pro Ball running back

Karin Smith, Olympic
javelin specialist

Amy Van Dyken,
Olympic swimmer
(gold medal)

Bonnie Warner, Olym-
pic luge specialist

Dominique Wilkins,
basketball player

Kristi Yamaguchi,
Olympic figure
skating (gold medalist)

Theresa Zabell,
Olympic athlete
(yachting)

Alex Zulle, Olympic
athlete (cycling)

ASTHMA MYTHS

Here is a list of commonly held myths about asthma. *Remember, all of them are false.* The facts are found in the noted chapters.

- Asthma is a psychological disease. (See chapter 1.)
- Asthma should prohibit children from physical activity—from playing on playgrounds to competitive sports. (See chapter 11.)
- Being treated in the emergency room or hospitalized is a normal part of having asthma. (See chapters 1 and 4.)
- Only the symptoms of asthma are treatable, and there is no treatment to control asthma and prevent symptoms or flares. (See chapter 5.)
- Certain breeds of dog are nonallergenic. (See chapter 3.)
- Inhaled corticosteroids or oral steroids (like prednisone) are the same as steroids taken and abused by athletes. (See chapter 5.)
- Nebulizers are better (stronger and more effective) than inhalers used with a spacer. (See chapter 6.)
- Asthma medicines are addictive. (See chapter 5.)
- Asthma medicines lose effectiveness over time, so it is better to take them only when absolutely needed. (See chapters 5 and 6.)
- Children or adults with asthma don't need to take medicine when they don't have symptoms. (See chapter 5.)
- Asthma flares occur suddenly and without warning. (See chapter 8.)

Useful Organizations

Allergy & Asthma Network: Mothers of Asthmatics
2751 Prosperity Avenue, Suite 150
Fairfax, VA 22031
Phone: 800-878-4403
Fax: 703-573-7794
www.aanma.org
Educational materials for patients, children, and schools; emotional support
to families who have children with asthma and allergies.

American Academy of Allergy, Asthma & Immunology (AAAAI)
611 East Wells Street
Milwaukee, WI 53202
Phone: 414-272-6071
E-mail info@aaaai.org
www.aaaai.org
Patient Information and Physician Referral Line: 1-800-822-2762 to request
printed information on allergies and asthma. Useful set of pamphlets called
"Tips" also available online. AAAAI cannot answer individual questions
relating to the diagnosis or treatment of allergies and asthma. AAAAI represents health professionals in research and treatment of allergic disease.

American Academy of Pediatrics (AAP)
141 Northwest Point Boulevard
Elk Grove Village, IL 60007
800-433-9016
www.aap.org
Public education resources.

American Association for Respiratory Care
11030 Ables Lane
Dallas, TX 75229-4593
972-243-2272
www.aarc.org

American College of Allergy, Asthma & Immunology (ACAAI)
85 West Algonquin Road
Suite 550
Arlington Heights, IL 60005
800-842-7777
www.allergy.mcg.edu
Health professionals' organization dedicated to patient care through research, advocacy, and public/professional education.

The American Lung Association
61 Broadway, 6th Floor
New York, NY 10006
212-315-8700 (national office)
800-LUNG-USA (for your local or regional office)
www.lungusa.org
Support groups, newsletters, asthma camp, asthma information.

Asthma and Allergy Foundation of America (AAFA)
1233 20th Street, NW, Suite 402
Washington, DC 20036
Phone: 800-7-ASTHMA or 202-466-7643
Fax: 202-466-8940
www.aafa.org
Private, nonprofit organization dedicated to finding a cure for asthma and allergic disease.

Clinical trials information
www.ClinicalTrials.gov

Food Allergy & Anaphylaxis Network (FAAN)
10400 Eaton Place, Suite 107
Fairfax, VA 22030
800-929-4040

www.foodallergy.org/
Public awareness, food allergy information, newsletter, videos, recipes/cookbook.

Healthy Kids: The Key to Basics
79 Elmore Street
Newton, MA 02159-1137
617-965-9637
www.information-engineer.com/kids/kidshp.htm
Educational planning for students with asthma and other chronic health conditions.

Journal of the American Medical Association: Asthma Information Center
www.ama-assn.org/special/asthma/
Peer-reviewed resources on asthma.

MedicAlert
800-432-5378
www.medicalert.org
MedicAlert bracelet or pendant; 24-Hour Emergency Response Center.

National Allergy Bureau
c/o American Academy of Allergy, Asthma and Immunology
Executive Office Center, Suite 600
2101 East Jefferson Street
Rockville, MD 20852
800-976-5536 or 877-922-4666
www.aaaai.org/nab/pollen.stm
Reports pollen and mold spore levels to media and the public.

National Asthma Education and Prevention Program (NAEPP)
301-251-1222
www.nhlbi.nih.gov/about/naepp
National Asthma Education and Prevention Program's Expert Panel Report 2:
Guidelines for the Diagnosis and Management of Asthma 1997
Asthma information for patients, schools, and the public; NAEPP materials include:
   Managing Asthma: A Guide for Schools
   Asthma Awareness Curriculum for the Elementary Classroom

Asthma and Physical Activity in School
Making a Difference: Asthma Management in the School (video)

National Education Association Health Information Network
1201 Sixteenth Street, N.W., Suite 521
Washington, DC 20036
202-822-7570
www.neahin.org

National Heart, Lung & Blood Institute Information Center
P.O. Box 30105
Bethesda, MD 20824-0105
www.nhlbi.nih.gov/guidelines/asthma/asthgdln.pdf

National Institute of Allergy and Infectious Diseases
301-496-4000
www.nih.gov/science/campus
Free pamphlets: dust allergy, mold allergy, pollen allergy, sinusitis.

National Jewish Medical and Research Center
1400 Jackson Street
Denver, CO 80206
800-222-LUNG
Asthma information; the only medical/research center in the United States
devoted entirely to respiratory, allergic, and immune system diseases.
www.njc.org

Pediatric/Adolescent Gastroesophageal Reflux Association, Inc. (PAGER)
301-601-9541
www.reflux.org

Pedipress, Inc.
Asthma peak flow diary and books such as: *Children with Asthma: A Manual for Parents,* by Thomas F. Plaut, M.D.
800-611-6081
www.pedipress.com

Support for Asthmatic Youth
1080 Glen Cove Avenue
Glen Head, NY 11545
516-625-5735

Index